# CONTROLLING HERPES NATURALLY

## *A Practical Guide to Treatment & Prevention*

Other Books by Michele Picozzi

*The Pocket Guide to Hatha Yoga*

*Yoga: The Perfect Companion*

# Controlling Herpes Naturally

Second Edition

*A Practical Guide to*
*Prevention & Treatment*

by

Michele Picozzi

Published by Southpaw Press

*Controlling Herpes Naturally:*
*A Practical Guide to Prevention & Treatment*



Electronically composed and printed in the
United States of America.



☙

Southpaw Press
1653 S. 2500 East
New Harmony, UT 84757-5083
www.herpesnomore.southpawpress.com
E-mail: support46@southpawpress.com

*Quantity discounts available.*

ISBN: 0-9658600-1-9

# Publisher's Note

The purpose of this book is to provide suggestions, information, resources and references for managing herpes outbreaks and related conditions. Individual results will vary.

We urge you to use common sense in all matters relating to your health. If any health problem persists or is accompanied by a high fever, it may indicate a serious condition, and you should seek medical attention.

The publisher intends to offer health information to help you cooperate with your health practitioner or medical doctor in your mutual pursuit for health. In the event that you use this information, without knowledge or approval from a health professional, it is your constitutional right to do so.

The publisher and author assume no responsibility. Neither the publisher nor author are affiliated with or receive compensation from any of the products or sources for products mentioned in this book.

In addition, as of press time, the URLs listed in the Resource section of *Controlling Herpes Naturally* refers to existing websites on the Internet. Users are advised to access the information found there at their own risk.

*This book is dedicated to people with herpes everywhere who have the will, courage and determination to take control of their health and well being.*

ଓ

# Table of Contents

ଓ

# Introduction to Second Edition

The herpes simplex (HSV) has outwitted man and medicine for centuries. A formidable foe, it exerts a tenacious and permanent hold deep within the human body.

After an initial episode, some individuals never see the evidence of herpesvirus on their skin again, while others have occasional bouts. Still, some carry on with chronic outbreaks.

While inherently not a fatal condition, there is no permanent cure for herpes. In the average healthy adult, herpes can be inconvenient, uncomfortable, and at times embarrassing because of the often-intimate nature of the condition and prevailing social stigma against sexually transmitted diseases (STDs).

The purpose of this book is to serve as a comprehensive self-help guide so you can better understand how the herpesvirus operates and for devising a strategy for keeping outbreaks under control.

In the following pages you will find many less expensive and safer alternatives to the prescription drugs currently available to treat the most common forms of herpes. Antiviral drugs, which suppress the replication of the herpesvirus, can cost from $95 to $225 monthly.

While these medicines can reduce the frequency of outbreaks, they are not nearly as effective at reducing the discomfort and duration of lesions. Side effects from these drugs are more likely to arise from continued use. Also, these medicines also don't mix well with drugs that treat heart conditions and blood sugar problems. Some people, particularly those with the oral form, find prescription medication don't relieve their symptoms.

On the other hand, there are many natural medicines that are safer, cheaper and more easily obtained that offer both short- and long term solutions to people with oral herpes referred to in this book by the acronym PWH and those with genital herpes will go by PWGH.

This book is a result of my education in treating my own oral herpes condition, which had become chronic as a young adult. The combination of my strong interest in alternative medicine, my desire not to suffer and to take control of my health propelled me to search for solutions. After some months of trial and error, I learned to control my outbreaks through yoga, diet, supplements and meditation. I have not had an outbreak anywhere on my face in years.

In the pages ahead, you will find many suggestions to chart your own wellness plan. Some methods will work quickly, but most will take some time to show results. Please be patient! There are great rewards to taking control of your health and doing the necessary work can bring lasting healing as well as a new understanding of yourself and your body. This kind of knowledge will serve you well for the rest of your life. I hope your will find the information helpful in your commitment to better health.

— *Michele Picozzi*

*Chapter 1*

# What's the Big Deal?

At a time when attention and research is focused on higher-profile illnesses involving impaired immunity such as HIV/AIDS, lupus, and chronic fatigue syndrome (CFS), there is another ailment that probably causes more human illnesses than any other. It hardly receives any media coverage or nearly as many research dollars as other diseases reflecting a state of impaired immunity. Yet it is just as common and infectious as it was before the AIDS outbreak. The ailment is herpes simplex.

Nearly 25 years has passed since herpes —primarily genital herpes— last created a stir in the U.S. Just as knowledge of acquired immune deficiency syndrome was just emerging. Before AIDS became a crisis, genital herpes was the most feared and dreaded sexually transmitted disease (STD). Millions, though, continue to experience painful recurrences of genital as well as facial herpes.

Herpes has been a curse of mankind since it surfaced more than 2,000 years ago. The virus comes by its name from the ancient Greek word *herpein* which means "to creep," a fitting description since diseases in ancient times were classified by their appearance.

Herpes actually is a collection of some 50 viruses. During the last 30 years, medical science has identified 8 different types of herpes that affect humans. The common forms of the herpes simplex virus, HSV-1 and HSV-2, and cause both primary and recurrent infections. HSV-1 is responsible for outbreaks appearing above the waist and most frequently on the face. However, outbreaks from HSV-1 can happen anywhere on the body. HSV-2 occurs below the waist, primarily on and around the genital area.

Despite the backseat herpes has taken in this age of considerably more life-threatening immune-related illnesses, reports from the Centers for Disease Control (CDC) find that approximately 1 in 3 people in the United States has been exposed to the highly contagious herpesvirus. Other studies say that 30 percent to 60 percent of U.S. children under age 10 have been exposed to the virus. Researchers at the University of California at Berkeley have estimated that 60 to 90 percent carry HSV-1, with the majority most likely picking up the infection during childhood. In 1997, the *New England Journal of Medicine* put the figure for Americans with facial herpes at 1 in 5.

Mostly these figures translate to approximately 30 million to 55 million Americans having experienced cold sores, fever blisters, genital blisters, shingles (a painful inflammation of the sensory nerves), chickenpox (HSV-3), infectious mononucleosis (caused by Epstein-Barr virus or HSV- 4), or cytomegalovirus (CMV or HSV-5) sometime in their lives.

According to a report issued by the CDC in May 2004, genital herpes affects at least 22 percent of the sexually active adults in the United States and infects between 200,000 and 400,000 each year. The condition affects about a total of 50 million Americans.

It wasn't always this way. Herpesvirus, as a medical condition of any consequence, was seldom mentioned in medical journals *before* 1966, about the time the sexual revolution took off. According to Stephen Sacks, M.D., the author of *The Truth About Herpes* (Gordon Soules, 1988), the most significant development in the increase of people contracting herpes is the introduction of the birth control pill. He writes, "As we left behind condoms and foam for the convenience of the IUD and the Pill, we left behind these unnatural, but effective barriers to infection."

Historically, genital herpes finds its way most often to Caucasians ranging in age from 15 to 29 years old, affecting more woman than men. According to Phyllis Stoffman, B.S.N., M.H. Sc., and author of *The Family Guide to Preventing and Treating 100 Infectious Illnesses* (John Wiley & Sons, 1995), most people will have a recurrence within six months of their first episode. By contrast, shingles will affect only 10 percent to 20 percent of the population, but the risk of an outbreak increases with age.

While the statistics mentioned here are only approximations of the actual number of people with herpesvirus (PWH) and apply only to the United States, HSV-1 and HSV-2 infection is common throughout the world. The high numbers of exposure and recurrences also reflect the insidiousness and remarkable staying power of herpes. Once contracted, HSV-1 (usually through the mouth from kissing or sharing the same utensils or towels) and HSV-2 (typically through the genitals or anus through sexual contact), the virus lives on in a dormant state in the body. After the initial infection, herpesvirus finds its way to groups of sensory nerve endings, called ganglia, located deep within the body at the base of the spinal cord or skull. Herpesvirus also is known to infect the fingers, eyes, and brain, often with more serious health consequences.

As yet, there is no vaccine to prevent contracting any form of herpesvirus. However, there are a number of natural healing agents when combined with lifestyle changes can dramatically increase the chances of controlling outbreaks as well as lessen the severity and duration of episodes.

The combined reality of the virus's prevalence in the general population and the reality of no known cure demand a proactive approach to the problem. This means doing what's necessary to keep both mind and body strong. This is the only reasonable and sensible alternative to controlling future outbreaks and further spreading the virus.

However, when working with the natural remedies in general and with those described here, they need time to work You also must be willing to experiment to find the right combination of remedies that will work for you. Good health requires balance and moderation.

PWH will find the most success in making positive changes in diet and lifestyle such as taking more or different types of supplements; taking up regular gentle exercise such as yoga, qigong or walking; getting more rest and taking time to truly relax, whether that means getting to bed earlier to take advantage of the body's healing cycle; spending more time alone or in nature; or listening to audio CDs or tapes for mental relaxation. The combination of these positive actions tempered with time, discipline and patience will help the body heal and strengthen itself to ward off future outbreaks. Good health requires a lifestyle that supports balance and moderation.

## Fact vs. Fiction: What You Should Know

***FICTION:*** If you don't have outbreaks with visible blisters or lesions present, you can't have herpes.

***FACT:*** Many who are infected with genital herpes have never had a visible blister or haven't recognized the symptoms, according to the latest research published in the New England Journal of Medicine. The study, conducted by the University of Washington, concluded that as many as 90 percent of people who have genital herpes don't know they have it.

Common symptoms of an initial infection with the herpes simplex-2 virus include:

- Flu-like symptoms such as stiff neck or pain in the area and sensitivity to light
- Reddening of small areas of the skin
- Other signs such as urinary tract infection in women, urethritis in men as well as genital burning or itching. Lesions that are internal or too small to see can cause any of these conditions.

***FICTION:*** Both oral herpes (cold sores) and genital herpes are spread only by skin-to-skin contact when an active or open sore is present.

***FACT:*** Passing the virus to another person occurs most often when you have an outbreak with visible sores. But both kinds of social herpes can be spread even when there is no lesion present by shedding skin that contains particles of the virus. This can occur even when taking prescription antiviral medication.

***FICTION:*** Oral herpes appears only on the mouth or face.

***FACT:*** You can be infected with oral herpes or HSV-1 in the genital area with the same symptoms associated with genital herpes.

Oral herpes can be transmitted during oral sex even if a condom is used. However, according to Peter Leone, MD, assistant professor of medicine, University of North Carolina (Chapel Hill), there's much less chance of passing the virus on via oral-to-genital transmission when the skin is healthy.

***FICTION:*** An examination by a medical professional during an active outbreak is the only sure way to know if you have herpes.

***FACT:*** That's one way of confirming the presence of the condition and so is examining a culture of an active lesion. There are two new methods to detect the presence of the virus, whether symptoms are present or not: the HerpesSelect ELISA kit and HerpeSelect Immunoblot kit. Both are available through private physician's offices and public health clinics.

*Chapter 2*

# Understanding Herpes

Herpes is classified in the medical world as a recurrent, highly contagious virus. As viruses go, herpes has earned a reputation for being one of the most persistent and pervasive viruses. And herpesvirus doesn't discriminate: It affects every animal species, in nearly every part of the world.

Generally speaking, viruses are considered by their very nature to be parasitic because they invade the host and then proceed to set up housekeeping in the host's cellular structure. Since viruses can't survive or duplicate on their own, they have the ability to wrap themselves in a protein "shell" to avoid detection by the immune system. In order to multiply, viruses are adept at confusing the immune system by changing its protein markers, shedding its protective protein sheath, and taking up residence in the host's cells. Then they go about their real work: mixing their DNA with the host cell's genetic code. Now the virus can really go to work, spreading through the body unchecked, invading more cells, and wearing down the body's defenses.

Scientists have identified herpesvirus as one of the most complicated viruses known to man. Some have gone as far as to call herpesvirus the ultimate parasite. Why such a strong and frightening label for a virus that is most commonly associated with the common cold? The simple explanation is that when herpesvirus has an opportunity to infect, it moves in, hides out in the human body and remains with an individual for life. So far despite all the great and wonderful advances in human health, herpesvirus has managed to evade a cure or pharmaceutical control.

At its core, herpesvirus carries DNA, the basic building block of life. Since herpesvirus lives inside a cell, antibodies that normally would fend off the virus from attack can't get to herpesvirus now inside a cell and destroy it. Part of what makes herpesvirus unique is that particles of the virus enter sensory nerve fibers where the infection is located, moving upward to where the nerve fiber begins. These are the body's pathways that carry the signals that allow the feelings of pain, touch, light, cold and so on. Sensory nerve fibers start from a small cluster of cells called sensory ganglion.

With facial or oral herpes (HSV-1), the virus remains in the ganglia located at the base of the skull known as the trigeminal ganglion. In genital herpes (HSV-2), the virus settles in to the sacral ganglia situated near the end of the spinal cord. Because of where the herpesvirus lives in the human body, it has proven to be a crafty invader, able to fend off the body's natural defenses.

When the virus sets out to resurface, herpesvirus travels down the path of the skin nerves and onto the skin, where it will wage war on skin cells to produce a new set of virus particles. If not stopped, painful ulcers or blisters surface on the skin. Because of the way herpesvirus behaves, it is considered a nerve-infecting virus and skin-blistering disease.

To devise an effective treatment to kill herpesvirus, scientists must formulate a drug that kills off the virus but not its host environment — the human body. Since there are so many viruses that plague humans, medical and pharmaceutical research tends to concentrate its efforts on developing antiviral drugs that will disable whole classes of viruses instead of one or two. Currently, three prescription drugs called "antivirals" — acyclovir (Zovirax), valcyclovir (Valtrex) and famciclovir (Famvir) — that treat oral and genital herpes.

## Common Types of Herpesvirus

While herpesvirus has been around for a very long time, understanding of it has been slow in coming. It wasn't until the '60s that medical researchers were able to identify and then label herpesvirus.

Herpesvirus encompasses about 50 different types of the virus, which all tend to look the same when placed under a high-powered microscope. The common denominator in this herpersvirus family is the viruses share an uncanny ability to remain in a dormant state within the human body until reactivated by some triggering event.

So far, medical science has isolated and identified 8 kinds of herpesvirus that affect people in any significant way.

Herpes simplex virus type 1 (HSV-1 or facial herpes, affecting the lips or face) and herpes simplex virus type 2 (HSV-2 or genital herpes, affecting the penis, anus, vagina, buttocks, and thighs) are the most well known and most frequently contracted. However, there is some debate in the medical community on whether or not HSV-1 and HSV-2 really are two different viruses. Much of the research indicates that they each represent a different strain, but are related. Others say that the herpesvirus that causes genital herpes may be the same the one that causes facial herpes but behaves differently on another part of the body. The common element of both these strains of herpesvirus is that they are extremely contagious, and spread by direct contact with the sores or the fluid they contain.

Varicella zoster, (which causes chickenpox and can reappear later as shingles), Epstein-Barr virus (identified as causing mononucleosis — "mono" or the "kissing disease" — and often found to be responsible for chronic fatigue syndrome), and cytomegalovirus (also associated with mononucleosis and more recently suspected in hepatitis) are classified as HSV-3, HSV-4, and HSV-5, respectively.

Discovered in 1986 by National Cancer Institute researchers, Epstein-Barr virus (EBV or HSV-6) also is considered a latent virus, hiding in the body's B cells, with the ability to reappear over and over again. Two years later, another herpesvirus, known as HBLV or HSV-7 was uncovered. It infects the cells in the body that manufacture virus antibodies and has been implicated as the cause of the fatigue that accompanies chronic fatigue syndrome. The recently discovered strains HSV-6 and HSV-7 have been found in people with chronic fatigue syndrome, while Type 6 has been observed in the T-cells of people who happen to have a variety of illnesses affecting their immune systems. In 1994, HSV-8 was first isolated from the lesions of Kaposi's sarcoma, a disease then commonly found in homosexual men with AIDS.

The two types of herpes simplex virus that infect most people are HSV-1, which is responsible for outbreaks appearing above the waist. HSV-1 appears on the body as cold sores or fever blisters on the lips or on areas of the face around the mouth and nose. There also is evidence that outbreaks of HSV-1 can happen anywhere on the body.

Genital herpes, caused predominantly by HSV-2, appears below the waist. Currently it is one of the most common sexually transmitted diseases, affecting millions of people alone in the United States. According to researchers, HSV-2 outbreaks seem to occur more frequently than HSV-1, particularly if the initial infection with the virus was a prolonged one. Men are thought to have 20 percent more recurrences than women, although the reason for this is not known.

The only good news about this cruel and persistent virus is seem to be that different types of herpes do not cause the same symptoms. Along the same vein, being infected with one type of herpes does not make infection with the others more likely.

**BUT having one form of herpes, particularly with oral and genital herpes, does not exclude the possibility of contracting another form of the virus.**

## Herpes Connection to Other Diseases

Scientists now believe that viruses, including herpes, are linked to illnesses that target the nervous, endocrine, and immune systems. Some recent reports have connected HSV-1 with Alzheimer's disease. Apparently this association applies only to people who also carry the apo E-4 gene. This gene, some researchers believe, is enough to predispose certain people to Alzheimer's. During the 1980's, evidence of connections between herpesvirus and other widespread illnesses began to accumulate. For instance, as many as 50,000 cases of CMV are contracted in the United States each year, with the 15- to 30-year-old age group the most seriously affected. CMV has the distinction of being least known of herpesviruses that affect humans, and some doctors consider it to be very dangerous. However, 80 percent of Americans over age 40 tests positively for CMV antibodies. Research now indicates that CMV, not EBV, causes mononucleosis and is transmitted through sexual contact.

In 1979, the *Archives of Internal Medicine* concluded that herpes simplex virus represents the great masquerader of our time. For example, herpesvirus has been implicated in chronic illnesses such as chronic fatigue syndrome, fibromyalgia, post polio syndrome, Lyme disease, lupus, and mild cases of multiple sclerosis.

By contrast, the *Journal of the American Medical Association* in 1992 reported that childhood herpes may actually lower an adult's risk of getting genital herpes and even AIDS. Some homeopathic doctors claim that childhood infections may be important in challenging the immune system. They theorize that viruses such as herpes serve to provoke and exercise the immune system and, ultimately, may be essential for disease prevention.

## How to Know When You Have Herpes

Whether it's a first episode or recurring one, you may feel unwell feeling as if you are coming down with a cold or the flu before you actually develop any outward signs of herpes. Typically, the symptoms that accompany an initial infection are the most severe you'll experience. Unfortunately, the most frequently noted symptoms also mimic flu symptoms or those associated with an upper respiratory infection, and include fever, swollen glands, chills, and fatigue. Eventually, blisters will occur on the mouth, face, or on or around the genitals or anus. It takes the body from 10 to 14 days to mount a defensive to rein in the infection..

Because the skin around the facial lips is a bit drier than the skin of the genitals, the blister stage appears more often here. Cold sores and fever blisters typically emerge at the slightly darker red border of the lips and the point where the thin mucous membrane of the mouth meets facial skin. Before HSV-1 becomes visible and erupts into a full-fledged sore, the affected patch of skin typically will first tingle, itch, then redden and appear puffy. As the blister draws more water to itself, it will grow larger and often the tiny blisters will run together. Then the blister or blisters will fill with a clear fluid or sometimes pus that will ooze and crust over and then vanish in about 7 to 10 days, leaving a darkened patch of skin that eventually disappears as well. Herpes sores that continually weep with pus should be examined by a medical professional and treated accordingly.

From the time the skin tingles or itches until the sores or blisters are completely healed, PWH should treat the situation as a highly contagious one, and take whatever precautions necessary so as not to infect others.

Skin that is overly moist or whose natural protection has been compromised by injury or trauma is an ideal setting for herpes transmission. This is because the virus enters the body through microscopic breaks or tears in the mucous membranes. Unfortunately, most areas of the body are likely territory for herpesvirus outbreaks. While the initial infecting bout with HSV-1 and HSV-2 frequently lasts longer and is considered more severe and painful, subsequent outbreaks that follow one after another can be equally painful.

For a certain diagnosis, an examination by a medical doctor is necessary. The characteristics of herpesvirus outbreaks are unique, and typically a visual examination of the affected area will confirm infection. Both HSV-1 and HSV-2 are considered external diseases of the skin. Genital herpes sometimes can be mistaken for syphilis or other diseases. In women, HSV-2 can settle on the cervix and therefore go undetected. There are several methods of laboratory testing including the staining of a smear, tissue culture, or blood test for antibodies. One specific blood test for diagnosing herpes is called the Western blot test. However, medical doctors consider a culture of the blisters or lesions as the benchmark for diagnosing HSV. For the most accurate testing, the culture must be obtained within the first 48 hours after symptoms appear.

Since *Controlling Herpes Naturally* was first published, two new tests have come on the market. Both are approved by the FDA and are offer an accuracy range for specificity and sensitivity between 89 and 100 percent. They are the HerpeSelect ELISA Kit and the HerpeSelect Immunoblot Kit, manufactured by Focus Technologies. Each looks for HSV1 and HSV2 antibodies, with results available in 1 to 2 weeks.

Many labs still used older tests accepted by the FDA because they are less expensive and widely available. However, they are not as reliable as the newer tests.

For an accurate confirmation on the type of HSV contracted, particularly with an initial infection, testing is advised. Dermatologists, the physicians who focus on diseases of the skin, are considered the medical specialists who treat people with herpes. Family doctors, general practitioners, internists, physician's assistants and nurse practitioners also are qualified to diagnose and treat HSV-1 and HSV-2.

### How Herpesvirus Works in the Body

Medical science considers herpes a slow virus. This class of viruses is characterized by long incubation periods, and is suspected as the cause of persistent and often neurological diseases, occurring long after the virus's initial contact.

After emerging from deep within the body, herpesvirus travels from one cell to another without ever leaving the cell's environment. The cell within the virus fuses with a neighboring cell by persuading it to build a series of bridges. Eventually a giant cell is created. Antibodies already circulating are sent to halt the spread of herpesvirus, but can't do much to defend against the invading virus since they can't easily get inside the cell to attack the virus. Meanwhile, herpesvirus is busy constructing bridges before its growth has progressed to the stage where the cell bursts open. It then hijacks human cells, instructing them to replicate, destroying healthy cells in the process.

### What Triggers Herpesvirus to Return

A variety of theories exist to explain what reactivates the dormant virus in our bodies, but exactly what causes about one-third of the people who have HSV-1 or HSV-2 to have recurrent outbreaks remains a mystery. However, there are certain situations that roust herpesvirus from its dormant state deep within the body's sensory nerve endings and send it on a return trip to the skin's surface.

While theories abound on what causes herpesvirus to reappear repeatedly, it really boils down to individual tolerance. What spurs herpesvirus into an active state can be of a physical or psychological nature or both? Emotional stress may be a strong factor for some, but for others it is unrelated. Elevated temperature at the site of the original herpes lesion caused by fever or exposure to UV-B rays (found in both sun and shade) often sets HSV-1 in motion for many, but not for all. The most commonly identified single triggers include eating nuts (particularly the ordinary peanut) or other foods with a higher percentage of the amino acid arginine (such as chocolate), exposure to sunlight, fever, being physically or emotionally run down (often these go together) or by experiencing chronic anxiety, worry, and even ambivalence. Women with compromised immune systems also may have recurrences that last longer or are more frequent or both.

Varicella zoster virus, which first manifests in childhood as chickenpox, can turn up again in adulthood as shingles. When VZV returns later in life, it typically is attributed to chronic stress, aging or impaired immune function. Opinion, though, varies on whether HSV-1 or HSV-2 has the highest incidence of recurrence. Again, subsequent outbreaks may depend on the individual, their general state of health, and their exposure to things and situations that can trigger an outbreak. While the debate goes on about rate of the virus's return, the general consensus among health professionals is that the immune system must function well and physical and mental stresses be kept at a manageable level if herpes is to be kept under control.

The following are the most common situations that have been found to trigger a herpesvirus outbreak:

- **Foods high in arginine.** Peanuts, almonds, seeds, chocolate, soybeans, gelatin, carob and coconut food with high arginine content. Almond paste, a common and often hidden ingredient in many baked goods, also can trigger a negative reaction in sensitive individuals. Onions, raw or fried, also should be avoided.
- **Ultraviolet light.** UV-B has been isolated as a trigger of facial herpes. Exposure to sunlight, particularly where and when rays are the strongest — beaches, mountains, lakes, and between 10 a.m. and 2 p.m.— should be avoided. PWH should use a sunscreen of SPF-15 or higher and wear a hat with a brim that covers the face. UV-B also has been linked to certain types of skin cancer.
- **Using known immunosuppressants.** Cigarettes, alcohol, recreational drugs, and refined sugar in all its many forms (especially high fructose corn syrup) all have been shown to suppress immune-system function. Consumers beware: *Chronic or excessive consumption of these substances puts the PWH at a distinct disadvantage in resisting future outbreaks.*
- **Increased internal acidity.** This can occur when stress levels are elevated or from eating foods that contribute to an over-acidic condition in the body. The most common offenders in this category are sugar, white bread, and other highly refined foods.
- **Menstruation**. While not conclusively proven because the pattern of recurrence can be intermittent, some women are more vulnerable to outbreaks before the start of their periods because of the significant hormonal changes taking place.
- **Strenuous physical activity.** This can tax the body's resources, depending upon current physical condition and stamina level. Recent studies have made a direct connection between reduced immune function and intense periods of exercise.

- **Trauma to the skin.** Recurrences are known to appear at the site of the injury, and routine dental procedures can trigger outbreaks for some PWH.
- **Increased moisture or friction.** Both conditions are present during sexual intercourse.
- **Seasonal changes.** Those with oral outbreaks are especially vulnerable when the body transitions from spring to summer and summer to fall. Traditional Chinese medicine maintains that major bodily organs undergo a period of change during seasonal transitions. For example, in the spring the liver is undergoes a cleaning out while during the transition from summer to fall the lungs are challenged.
- **Illness or disease.** With the immune system fighting off other predators, it can become taxed, giving the latent herpesvirus an opportunity to reappear. It comes as no surprise that the common cold is one of the most precipitating factors to an outbreak of facial herpes.
- **Stress, stress, and more stress.** There are theories that suggest that psychological stress itself alone can arouse the dormant herpesvirus all by itself. The #1 factor responsible for repeated and frequent outbreaks is stress, says Dr. Richard Hamilton in *The Herpes Book* (J.P. Tarcher, 1980). His experience with hundreds of PWH has demonstrated this theory beyond a shadow of a doubt. Emotional stress does two things to the body. First, it can suppress the body's natural antiviral agent, interferon; and then even simple, everyday stress can hinder the body's ability to make the antibodies it needs to fight any type of infection. How psychological stress affects PWH will be discussed in more detail in chapter four.

## How Herpes Communicates with the Body

As decidedly invasive and persistent as herpesvirus is, it often sends specific signals warning it is about to surface on the body. The medical term for this phenomenon is *prodrome* which is defined as the warning the body send to the brain to signal an impending attack before the main set of symptoms appear. More than 50 percent of PWH say they experience one or more prodromes, or internal warnings, before an outbreak. These signs and sensations are thought to happen in 90 percent of recurrences and typically occur at the exact site of previous infections.

**Recognizing the "on-alert" symptoms when they first occur can be a PWH's most valuable asset in controlling outbreaks and spreading herpesvirus.**

One theory to explain prodromes finds that as herpes viral particles move from the ganglia toward the skin cells, they may irritate the nerves slightly and thereby create the prodromal sensations. Another hypothesis supposes that as these affected cells swell, die, and disintegrate, they cause the itching and tingling that serve as warning of an impending herpesvirus outbreak.

Experts agree that skin sensitivity is the most noticeable early warning people with HSV-1 and HSV-2 routinely experience — specifically, tingling, itching, or stinging sensations near the place on the skin where the initial or previous herpesvirus outbreaks occurred. These prodromes can last from a few minutes to hours or up to a couple of days.

Prodromes vary in variety and intensity from person to person. By becoming aware of the internal signs or signals your body is sending, it is possible to help minimize the length and discomfort of an outbreak or stop it altogether. Equally important to remember is to take precautions against infecting others at this stage. Until recently, the point at which herpesvirus can be passed from one person to another was undefined. Laboratory tests have now demonstrated that contagious virus particles can be shed and transmitted at the outset of warning sensations, before the development of any blisters. It would be unwise to ignore the overwhelming evidence that exists in spreading the virus when no blisters are present.

**Since herpesvirus is spread only by direct, physical contact, the wise, responsible, and kind course of action is to avoid all close physical contact — kissing, intercourse, sharing towels, toothbrushes, lip balm, etc. — at the first sign of any internal warning sensation or prodrome.**

The early warning signs of an outbreak most often reported by PWH include:

- *Crawling* — the sensation that something is crawling or creeping beneath the skin.
- *Heat* — a warm throbbing at the site.
- *Invisible scratch* — feeling as if there were a slight abrasion on the skin, but none is visible.
- *Isolated sensations* — sometimes similar to the tingling or pins-and-needles sensation described later in this list, but restricted to a different and seemingly unrelated part of the body. For example, one PWGH reported feeling a specific sensation in her foot preceding a herpes outbreak.
- *Itchiness* — the feeling that something is on or just below the skin or that a rash is on the verge of emerging.
- *Malaise and general fatigue* — the general complaint of feeling "sick and tired" often signals an attack, but

is nonspecific. That is, no one part of the body feels particularly bad, but simply feeling a general sense of malaise.

- *Muscular aches and pains* — the muscles near the nerve paths involved in the migration of virus particles sometimes ache or throb with a dull pain. In the case of oral herpes, PWH sometimes report that their cheeks and jaw muscles ache.
- *Neuralgia* — an impending viral attack is sometimes characterized by pain, usually mild, but sometimes quite sharp, radiating through the lower back or down the legs or throughout the planes of the face.
- *Phantom inflammation* — the area feels inflamed, and perhaps is even warm to the touch, yet is not visibly so.
- *Pins and needles* — as if a small patch of skin had "fallen asleep," much as a limb in a cramped position will lose sensation and then "come back to life."
- *Pressure* — the sensation that something is pushing under the skin or pressing up against the surface.
- *Prickly sensations* — like tiny jabs in the skin.
- *Slight surface aching*— on or near the site of past outbreaks.
- *Swollen glands* — lymph glands swell when an infection takes hold thus stimulating the immune system into action. Although this symptom usually accompanies the primary or initial attack of herpesvirus, many patients report swollen glands as a prodromal symptom. Perhaps the immune system anticipates the impending viral infection and begins to gear up against it, with increasing activity in the lymph nodes.
- *Tingling* — an almost ticklish feeling, sometimes as if there were a slight vibration beneath the skin.
- *Touch sensitivity* — the skin feels sore or as if a pimple were about to erupt.

☾ *Twitchiness* – as if there were a slight spasm or twitch beneath the skin.

Prodromes almost always mean that the HSV has been reactivated within the body, whether or not outward physical signs such as blisters appear. Sometimes the course of the recurrence can be short-circuited, resulting in reddening of the skin, but no blisters. The reasons for this aren't clear. False prodromes, as they are called, are known to happen more frequently in PWH who take regular doses of acyclovir.

## Genital Herpes and Pregnancy

Women who have genital herpes are encouraged to inform their doctor of their condition as soon as they learn they are expecting. Critical problems may arise with herpes and pregnancy that can be avoided if precautions are planned for in advance.

The medical profession takes this situation very seriously as an active outbreak at the time of delivery can pass on virus to a newborn if the baby passes through the birth canal. The journal *Sexually Transmitted Diseases* (2005) reports that one in four mothers has genital herpes, with many of them not knowing they have it, and can pass the virus on to their babies.

While transmission of the virus from the mother to the newborn delivered through birth canal is considered low (less than 0.1 percent in the U.S.), contacting HSV2 can cause severe brain damage or death. Left untreated up to 85 percent of neo-natal herpes cases can be fatal.

To minimize the risk of infecting a newborn, C-sections or Cesareans are performed routinely when the mother either has frequent genital herpes outbreaks or has an active infection when labor begins.

A woman who has contracted the virus before becoming pregnant passes herpes antibodies to the fetus that protects the unborn baby from becoming infected with the virus. After birth, though, the baby loses this protection as he or she begins to develop its own immune system.

For women who do not have genital herpes, but whose partners already have or suspect they carry HSV2, the Center for Disease Control and Prevention advises these women to avoid intercourse and oral sex during their third trimester. The agency also reports that women who contract the herpesvirus for the first time while pregnant have a greater risk for passing the virus to their babies because the mother does not have time to build up antibodies.

Also, because of their immature immune systems, infants are particularly at risk for getting herpes. People with oral or facial herpes should avoid kissing a baby until their skin has healed completely.

*Chapter 3*

# Conventional & Alternative Treatments

### *What Traditional Medicine Offers to Control the Virus*

In 1972, approximately six years after the rapid rise in incidences of genital herpes, researchers at the pharmaceutical giant then called Burroughs-Wellcome Co. (now Glaxco-Wellcome) developed acyclovir. Clinical trials for the drug known as BW248-U were conducted from the late 1970s through the early 1980s at the University of Seattle, Emory University, and University of Vermont. The results were encouraging and in March 1982 the FDA approved acyclovir for sale as a prescription drug under the brand name Zovirax.

It is composed of a synthetic analog of the chemical deoxyguanosine that occurs naturally and is required by cells to produce DNA. Acyclovir works by subverting the viral genes; not by killing them off, but by exchanging live "bullets" with "blanks." Since herpesvirus needs a certain enzyme to replicate, acyclovir fools the virus into using it instead of the proper enzyme. Once herpesvirus accepts the fake enzyme into its genetic structure, the virus can't reproduce itself because technically it is genetically incomplete. While the drug acts to stop replicating the virus, it can't spread to otherwise healthy cells.

Since acyclovir attacks only the infected cells, it doesn't disturb cells unaffected by herpesvirus. Healthy cells don't contain thymidine kinase and therefore won't seek out acyclovir. What makes acyclovir so specific in the treatment of herpesvirus is that the particular enzyme it imitates is found only in human cells that have been attacked by herpesvirus.

Acyclovir (Zovirax) is classified as an antiviral drug and comes in ointment, capsules, liquid, and IV form. It is most often prescribed for HSV-1, HSV-2, shingles and chickenpox. At this time, a generic form of the drug does not exist. Typical treatment protocol calls for dosing with acyclovir at the first sign of a prodrome or lesion, with dosage varying from two doses of 200 mg, 3 times a day or 1 to 5 times a day for 7 consecutive days. However, in severe cases, long-term dosage extends from 1 to 3 years. Maintenance therapy to prevent recurrences typically consists of two to three daily doses of 200 mg. Recurrences are common after when the acyclovir therapy is stopped, but with less frequency than before.

Acyclovir, however, can't be counted on to prevent either the latent infection state or recurrent infections. Clinical studies have not shown any conclusive proof that acyclovir can act to prevent the virus from moving into the latent or dormant stage even with early usage of the drug. Also important to remember is that acyclovir has no effect on the virus hiding in the nerve ganglia and, does not eliminate the virus from the body.

Possible side effects of acyclovir include itching or burning of the skin, nausea, vomiting, anorexia, depression, tremors, headache, dizziness, vertigo, general weakness, blood in the urine and allergic skin reactions. Side effects of the drug may increase if taken with cyclosporine (an immunosuppressant), penicillamine, and some cancer drugs. In addition, taking this drug in combination with interferon and methotrexate (used for psoriasis, cancer, and rheumatoid arthritis) may affect the nervous system. Physicians do not recommend routine use of acyclovir by patients with recurrent genital herpes. Approximately 20 percent of PWH fail to find relief through acyclovir, and some people with AIDS have shown resistance to acyclovir.

Other popular prescription drugs for HSV-1 and HSV-2 include:

*Valtrex (valacyclovir)* — is the second often prescribed drug treatment for genital herpes, and is also made and sold by Glaxo Wellcome. An initial clinical trial of Valtrex indicated that healing took nine days on average, with the accompanying pain persisting for a minimum of five days. In addition, the average amount of time for viral shedding to cease was three days. Valtrex also is reported requiring two doses daily compared with five for Zovirax (acyclovir).

Side effects are similar to those associated with Zovirax. The effects of Valtrex can increase dangerously if taken with benemid and cimetidine (Tagamet, Tagamet HB).

*Famvir* — treats genital herpes exclusively and is manufactured by SmithKline Beecham Pharmaceuticals. Side effects include headache, migraine, burning sensation on the skin, nausea, diarrhea, vomiting, intestinal gas, abdominal pain, fatigue, skin rash and menstrual cramps.

*Denavir* (penciclovir) — the first drug specifically approved for cold sores was introduced in May 1997 by SmithKline Beecham. It is sold as a topical cream. A study in the Journal of the American Medical Association demonstrated Denavir's ability to provide relief from pain, improve healing by one day and shorten the time the virus was contagious. According to research physician

Spotswood Spruance of the University of Utah, people with more severe infections probably experience better results. In the trial, the most frequently reported side effects reported were headaches and skin irritation.

## The Best Alternative Treatments for Herpes

### Herpanacine®

When a trial formula of vitamins, herbs, and amino acids showed positive results on a group patients with recurrent viral and bacterial skin infections, Dr. Wayne Diamond, a naturopath and psychologist practicing in suburban Philadelphia introduced this new formula, marketed under the brand name Herpanacine®, to the public in 1990.

A synchronistic formula, Herpanacine®'s 10 ingredients work together to achieve maximum absorption by the body to provide relief from recurring viral and bacterial infections.

The supplement consists of lysine (to suppress multiplication of herpesvirus); beta-carotene (to cleanse skin layers and the immune system of toxins); L-tyrosine (to balance the nervous system); vitamin E (to purify dermal tissue of toxins and to increase stamina); selenium (to reduce viral cell growth); dandelion root (to reduce excessive acidity in blood and skin and to support liver function); sarsaparilla (to disperse toxins from blood); and astragalus, lingustrum, and echinacea (to reduce viral and bacterial cells in blood and skin layers and to boost immunity).

"I think of it as skin support system from the inside out," says Diamond, explaining further that Herpanacine's purpose is to balance the body's overall chemistry, cleanse the skin's layers, build up immunity so the body is able to overcome future outbreaks.

According to materials published by Diamond-Herpanacine Associates, Herpanacine® has a cumulative effect on both the nervous and immune systems. Results typically are seen between the second and sixth months of taking the supplement on a daily basis. The longer it is taken, the company advises, the more effective it can be in contributing to overall well being. Some users also may experience increased energy and stamina.

*Suggested uses:*

- For severe conditions: Take 3 capsules in the morning and 3 more in the afternoon.
- For less serious conditions or when improvement occurs: take 2 capsules in the morning; repeat in the afternoon.
- For maintenance after condition shows improvement: Take 1 capsule in the morning and 1 in the afternoon.

*Note: Herpanacine® should always be taken with food.*

**Lysine**

Lysine has distinguished itself as the primary natural remedy for preventing and treating herpesvirus. Many practitioners, traditional medical and alternative, consider this amino acid to be the definitive link to controlling outbreaks. Lysine is one of more than 20 amino acids that make up the body's proteins and it is one of the eight essential amino acids. Amino acids (which really aren't acids in the conventional sense) are the raw materials your body needs to grow and repair itself. Since amino acids are life's essential building blocks, every cell in our bodies requires them. Viruses also need amino acids to reproduce.

Stephen Cooter, Ph.D., author of *Beating Chronic Illness,* writes that known lysine- deficiency symptoms, caused in part by a high-arginine diet and without viral complications, resemble the basic weakness and fatigue problems that are common symptoms in many chronic illnesses and believes that lysine is one possible way of rejuvenating the immune system.

Lysine also is necessary in forming antibodies so the immune system can fend off whatever invaders challenge it. It nourishes the blood and aids in the formation of antibodies by building immunity. Since the body does not make lysine it is essential to eat enough protein or take supplements.

Interest in lysine as a treatment for herpesvirus started with when lysine was added to a virus culture and researchers noticed the amino acid could inhibit viral growth. Further research found that by varying the ratio of amino acids in human cells, growth patterns of virus in those cells could be altered. The ratio that changed the most was the relationship of lysine to arginine, another naturally occurring amino acid. When there was more lysine than arginine, viral activity slowed. When there was more arginine than lysine, viral activity increased. In *Amino Acids in Therapy,* Dr. Leon Chaitow concluded that diets rich in lysine or aided by supplementation could thwart the replication of herpesvirus. Dietary choices, he observed, can either encourage or discourage viral-related disease.

Since a high ratio of lysine to arginine seemed to inhibit growth of herpesvirus, researchers theorized that viral production in PWH might be slowed to the point of decreasing symptoms. Several studies on lysine and herpesvirus conducted over the last 15 years have produced very encouraging results such as those listed below:

- A study in Denmark concluded that when PWH took a prophylactic daily dose of lysine over a long period of time, it was more effective than taken when the patients experienced prodromal signs signaling a possible recurrence of herpesvirus.

- In a clinical study conducted at Indiana University, 250 patients with cold sores were given lysine in dosages ranging from 312 to 1,200 mg. Only two showed no improvement, while 248 did. The researchers concluded that lysine was a definite positive factor in recovering from an outbreak of HSV. The scientists also learned from their subjects that their pain was reduced, lesion spread was halted and healing was speeded up.
- Other reports say that lysine helps other herpes-related diseases including Bell's palsy (a type of facial paralysis) and Ménierè's disease (a disorder of the inner ear).

Foods rich in lysine are chicken, turkey, beef, lamb, fish, milk, cheese, beans, mung bean sprouts and brewer's yeast. Foods with inadequate amounts of lysine include most grains, rice, wheat, oats and millet. Pork, though it has more arginine and lysine, probably should be avoided by PWH who have frequent outbreaks or those with weakened immune systems. Also, pigs are exposed to many viral and fungal infections are thought be transmittable to humans.

Lysine also helps build resistance to bacteria and promotes a general feeling of well- being. When taking lysine or other amino acids, it's best to take them on an empty stomach and supplemented with vitamins C and $B_{6.}$

However, lysine by itself may not be as effective as a preventive tool. This is the opinion of Dr. Wayne Diamond, a naturopath and psychologist, who created Herpanacine®, a dietary supplement for viral and bacterial skin infections. His research argues that lysine use alone can be inconsistent as a prevention tool, and for some PWH, lysine doesn't work at all.

In addition, best-selling author Andrew Weil, M.D., finds lysine to be more effective against oral herpes (HSV-1) than genital herpes (HSV-2).

## Other Fortified Lysine Supplements

*Super Lysine Plus+*™ is probably the oldest herb-and-vitamin formula for herpes on the market and is manufactured by Quantum. Lysine is the primary ingredient in the formula and is fortified by garlic, echinacea, vitamin C, propolis, licorice, goldenseal root and shiitake mycelium *Super Lysine Plus+*™ is available in tablet and extract form.

*Lysine Herbal*® by Zand comes in capsule form and contains 500 mg of lysine, magnesium, zinc, vitamin $B_{12}$, folic acid, and selenium in a base of Chinese and Western herbs to support immune function.

## Essential Herbs

- **Echinacea** – serves as a multipurpose formula with antibiotic, immune enhancing and antiseptic properties that regulates the glandular system and is cleanses the internal body. The root extract believed to show interferon-like activity and antiviral action against the flu, herpes, and other viruses. When tincture form is held in the mouth for several minutes, echinacea will produce a numbing effect.
- **Goldenseal –** is a natural antibiotic, sometimes called Russian penicillin, and antiseptic. It regulates liver function and supports glandular function. Reputed to cleanse and dry the mucous membranes.

- ☾ **Astragalus** — stimulates the immune system and white blood cell levels. Improves resistance to illness. Also restores harmony between kidneys and spleen and supports liver function.
- ☾ **Eleutherococcus (formerly known as Siberian Ginseng)** — excellent overall tonic for increasing energy and enhancing physical and mental well being. Strengthens the adrenal glands, supports the nervous and cardiovascular system and boosts resistance to stress and infection.
- ☾ **Licorice** — acts as an anti-inflammatory and has antiviral properties. Protects the liver and supports adrenal function. The glycyrrhizic acid in licorice suggests enhanced interferon production. Individuals who have high blood pressure should use caution when taking licorice extract supplements because licorice can cause the body to retain sodium and lose potassium
- ☾ **Alfalfa** — supports central nervous system function.
- ☾ **Burdock** — cleanses liver and supports immune function.
- ☾ **Dandelion** — cleanses liver and supports health of the myelin sheath of the nerves.
- ☾ **Red Clover** — acts as a general tonic for the nerves.
- ☾ **St. John's Wort** — functions as an antidepressant and improves energy and appetite. Hypericin, one of the active ingredients of St. John's Wort, according to laboratory test results published in Antiviral Research (1991), may help kill HSVI and HSVII.

*Note: Alternative health care practitioners suggest taking these herbs for short intervals, one to two weeks at a time.*

## Herbs to Relax the Nerves

The central nervous system is closely related to the workings of the immune system. The digestive system is aligned with the immune system. Between them, information is constantly passed back and forth. These interdependencies of these body mechanisms are important to keep in mind when looking to heal the body of a chronic condition such as herpesvirus. In many instances the nervous system needs to be repaired first before immune function can be resorted. A few herbs and grains are considered tonics for the nerve tonics since they exert a beneficial affect on the nervous system.

Common nervines include:

- ☾ Oats (tonic or in whole food form) — known for soothing the nervous and digestive systems.
- ☾ St. John's Wort — an excellent restorative for calming the nervous system. (Suggested dosage is 20 drops, 3 times daily.) Note: Avoid overexposure to sunlight while taking this supplement.
- ☾ Valerian — often called the herbal Valium.
- ☾ Passion flower — soothes central nervous system.
- ☾ Skullcap —calms nervous system, cleanses liver.
- ☾ Peppermint and chamomile — are the most commonly used herbal relaxants and make soothing teas. When heated, they release compounds that have a tranquilizing effect on the body.
- ☾ Kava kava — in addition to relieving symptoms of anxiety and insomnia, it also may relieve pain and act as an anti-viral and antibacterial agent.

A physician practicing in Southern California prescribes 750 mg of the amino acid GABA (gamma-aminobutyric acid) 3 times daily, after meals to calm the nerves. Also, magnesium (200-400 mg daily) may help balance out some of the damage caused by stress as it blocks the damaging effects of adrenaline.

## Other Helpful Herbs

- *Cascara Sagrada* – contains the active ingredient *anthraquinones* which some consider to have the ability to kill herpes simplex, reports Heniz Rosler, Ph.D., associate professor of medicinal chemistry at the University of Maryland School of Pharmacy in Baltimore. Use product labeled U.S.P. to make sure it has been aged for a least a year. Bark that has not been aged correctly contains chemicals that can cause violent diarrhea and severe intestinal cramps. Product labeled U.S.P. ensures at least a year's worth of aging. This herb is traditionally used as a laxative and should be avoided if you are pregnant or have ulcers, ulcerative colitis, irritable bowel syndrome, hemorrhoids, or other gastrointestinal conditions.
- *St. John's Wort* – New York University researchers have found the herb has dramatic action against the type of virus that causes AIDS. It contains antiviral, antibacterial, and anti-inflammatory chemicals. It is especially recommended for topical applications and internal use when cold sores are the result of a feeling of overall exhaustion.
- *Tarragon* – contains caffeic acid, an ingredient that could prevent herpes as well as cancer and the flu. For a synergistic effect, drink lemon balm tea with an added teaspoon of dried tarragon. Brew for 10 to 15 minutes; drink up to 3 cups a day. Both herbs possess antiviral activity.

## External Alternative Treatments

- *Aloe vera* — is a classic natural remedy because of its superior ability to heal and soothe the skin (it contains $B_1$, $B_2$, $B_6$ and C) plus excellent antiviral properties. A study conducted by the University of Maryland (Baltimore) Dental School found that applying pure aloe vera gel or a lip balm with at least a 50 percent concentration of the plant reduced blister pain and speeded up healing. The most potent form available is directly from the plant itself. Pieces of the stalk can be sliced off when needed, with the clear, fleshy part applied directly to the skin. These plants are easy to grow; requiring bright light and little water.
- *Myrrh* — in tincture form it acts as an antiseptic and anti-inflammatory effect on the mucous membranes, reduces inflammation, and speeds healing. Contains tannins.
- *Lemon balm* — also contains beneficial tannins that are useful in speeding healing and reducing pain. A European study concluded that people with cold sores or genital herpes who applied a cream containing lemon balm extract five times daily cut the healing rate for lesions nearly by half. This herb also makes for a soothing and delicious hot tea.
- *Tannins* — are naturally occurring substances primarily found in most black and green teas, red wines and myrrh and contain a variety of antioxidants that help heal herpes lesions. Simple remedies for healing herpes lesions include applying a cold wet bag of Earl Grey (bergamot) tea or congealed red wine.

**Red Wine Remedy**

**Set aside a small amount of red wine, enough to cover the bottom of the glass. Let it stand overnight. In the morning, the wine will have congealed into a concentrated form. Take a cotton swab and dab directly on sores.**

## Other Helpful Supplements

### *Thymus Extract*

Chronic infections caused by viruses, allergies, or autoimmune diseases can be traced to thymus gland functioning under par. Repetitive infections can weaken thymus function.

The theory behind glandular extract therapy is similar to homeopathy where like cures like. As a healing technique, it dates back to the ancient Greeks. Today, glandular extracts are commonly given to support the function of the thyroid, adrenal, pituitary, pancreas, liver and spleen.

Active ingredients in glandular extracts include peptides, enzymes, vitamins, minerals, hormone precursors and natural lipid factors.

Naturopath and prolific author Michael T. Murray recommends a thymus extract in these situations to normalize the ratio of T-helper cells to suppressor cells and restore immune function.. He suggests buying thymus preparations from reputable brands that contain about 750 mg of crude peptide fraction.

Enzymatic Therapy makes two excellent products that contain predigested thymus fractions. *ThymuPlex*® combines thymus extracts with a handful of immune-boosting antioxidants and herbs together with lysine. *Thymulus*®

contains thymus extract with 250 mg of astragalus that supports immune function and boosts resistance to illness by enhancing the production of T-cells, the white blood cells that fight viral and bacterial infections.

Glandular extracts should only be used for a short times as the thymus gland will continue to function on its own after getting a "jump-start" from the corresponding glandular extract.

***Colostrum and Lactoferrin***

These dietary supplements are obtained from first milk of nursing cows and are thought to support immunity while offering antibacterial, antiviral, antifungal and anti-inflammatory properties. These claims have been supported only by studies done on animals and in laboratories. So far there are no reliable studies of colostrums and lactoferrin on humans. However, researchers do agree that both supplements have iron-binding properties that support the immune system in fighting off bacteria that needs iron to replicate.

Those allergic to cow's milk as well as pregnant and nursing women should avoid both these supplements.

***Monolaurin***

An antiviral supplement used to treat infections such as measles and HIV, monolaurin disables bacteria, yeast, fungi as well as viruses. It shows great promise in preventing future outbreaks of all types of herpes.

A nontoxic dietary supplement made from lauric acid (a fatty acid found in breast milk) and glycerin, the supplement is sold under the brand name Lauricidin and comes in miniature pellets.

Monolaurin is thought to work by pulling the plug on fat-coated viruses such as herpes by sending fluids to penetrate the lipids and phospholipids in their coverings for the purpose of dissolving viral particles.

According to Dr. Andrew Weil, dosage for Lauricidin must be determined individually and is best taken under a physician's supervision. Information on his website (www.drweil.com) recommends starting with a low dose of 1.5 grams once or twice daily for 1 or 2 weeks to be followed with an increased dose of 3.0 grams taken 1 or 2 times daily, if the supplement is well tolerated and there is improvement. Suggested maintenance dose is 3.0 grams 2 to 3 times daily.

Additional information about dosing is available through Jon Kabara, M.D., the physician and researcher who developed monolaurin, when placing an order at his website (www.lauricidin.com).

### *Diethyl Ester*

Another well-documented remedy and also recommended by Dr. Andrew Weil. Suggested use is one drop of diethyl ester placed daily on a lesion. Normally inhaled, DE is an anesthetic and can be mildly irritating to the skin. According to Dr. Weil, the substance promotes both drying and healing. Diethyl ester can be obtained from a pharmacist and may be mixed with aspirin.

## Chinese Patent Medicines

Chinese medicine offers a wide array of plant-based patent medicines to treat both symptoms and underlying internal imbalance.

These formulas are especially effective for self-limiting health conditions such as the common cold, herpes outbreaks, urinary tract infections, insomnia, anxiety and indigestion, to name a few. Many of these combination herbal remedies have been used for thousands of years and often come in colorful packages.

Chinese patent medicines aim to stop the progress of a simple illness before it becomes more serious condition requiring prescription drugs that often have unpleasant side effects, can be expensive and tend not to resolve the underlying condition.

The Chinese patent medicines suggested here to quell herpes outbreaks come in small, dark round pills often referred to as teapills. Typically, teapills consist of several herbs cooked together until a highly concentrated mixture is formed and rolled into tiny balls finished with a protective glaze. Sometimes the same formulas come in conventional coated tablets, depending on the manufacturer.

Generally, these formulas imported from China are safe to use. However, from time to time, concerns about their safety have been raised since heavy metals or drugs have been known to be added by some manufacturers to certain formulas. To ensure safety, buy only reputable brands such as Plum Flower (sold primarily by Mayway Corporation based in Oakland, California), Golden Flower or Lanzhou Foci.

Each formula carries dosage instructions and most call for 8 pills, 3 times daily. This may sound like a large dose, but since these are herbs and not concentrated pharmaceuticals they can be safely taken in larger doses. A licensed acupuncturist or an herbalist who has studied Chinese herbs should be consulted for best results. Some Internet sellers of Chinese patent medicines offer brief telephone or email consultations to their customers.

- ☾ **Long Dan Xie Gan (Gentanae Teapill)** — This is one of the most popular formulas for treating outbreaks and treats a wide range of inflammatory conditions. Take at the first sign of an outbreak and continue to speed healing. Subdues liver fire.

- ☾ **Bi Xie Sheng Shi Wan** (Subdue the Dampness) — Clears damp heat.
- ☾ **Shen Qi Da Bu Wan** — Traditionally prescribed for weak immunity, fatigue and lack of appetite.
- ☾ **Bai Hi Tang** (White Tiger) — Used for heat signs such as fever and cold sores.
- ☾ **Huang Lien Shang Ching Pien** — Commonly used for mouth infections as well as bronchitis and skin rashes. If causes diarrhea, discontinue use. Not for use during pregnancy.

## Homeopathy

Homeopathy can be helpful in relieving and stalling future outbreaks of herpesvirus. This system of healing is based on the theory that "like cures like." Remedies are taken in minute doses to help the body do what it wants to do: heal itself. Samuel Hahnemann introduced homeopathy 200 years ago in Germany. Currently, there are more than 2,000 homeopathic preparations, with 200 to 300 of these considered polycrest formulas, the most popular remedies.

Dana Ullman, M.P.H., an author of several popular books on homeopathy, says that symptoms of illness not only represent a sign of illness, but also the body's best efforts to try to defend and heal itself. From this perspective, treatments such as many conventional drugs that seek to stop, inhibit, or control these efforts are ignoring the body's inherent wisdom and suppressing its ability to heal itself. He also cautions that self-treatment of herpes with homeopathic medicines will commonly get rid of the eruptions quickly, but professional, constitutional care is recommended if you want to reduce the frequency or intensity of eruptions and potentially eliminate them altogether.

In selecting a homeopathic remedy, pick the one that describes your most primary symptoms. The most often recommended homeopathic remedies for HSV-1 and HSV-2 include *Nitricum muriaticum, Sepia, Graphites, Rhus Toxicodendron,* and *Dulcamara.*

## How to Take Homeopathic Remedies

Homeopathic remedies come in potencies labeled 6, 12 or 30 with either and "X" or "C" next to the number. Remedies with a lower number indicate that it works more physically and for a shorter period of time. The same applies for the "X" scale of potencies. Higher numbers and those marked to the "C" scale work a little longer and deeper in your system. These remedies can be used less often.

Whatever potency you choose (30X being the most commonly suggested), take frequently (every 1 to 2 hours) during the early stages of an outbreak. When symptoms subside, reduce frequency to 1 to 3 times daily.

Breakout will likely lessen in frequency and intensity if homeopathic remedies are taken during consecutive flare-ups. This is due to the intense curative effects of these remedies.

When improvement occurs, discontinue the remedy or if there is no noticeable after 48 hours, consider trying another remedy.

**For acute eruptions of herpes on the mouth:**

- *Rhus tox* (poison ivy) is indicated when the symptoms either start at night or are worse at night and manifest as small fluid-filled blisters that itch or cause pain and eventually crust over. Blisters typically form around the lips, chin or nose. Individual may be sensitive to cold and dampness.
- *Natur muriaticum* (sodium chloride) treats eruptions that start or are worse in the daytime and when cracks appear at the corner or the mouth or below the corner and swelling that occurs in the center of the lips. Blisters are either large and clear or appear as clusters of small, watery blisters. These eruptions could be triggered by sun or hot weather. The mouth tends to be dry and the individual affected may be thirsty. It is most useful in the early phase of an outbreak and when emotional upset is present.
- *Hepar sulphur* (calcium sulphide) is helpful for eruptions around the mouth and lips or around the eyes and can be extremely sensitive to touch or cold. Use when sores have become infected with yellow pus.
- *Sepia* (cuttlefish ink) also treats outbreaks around the lips, corners of the mouth and especially around the nose. Person affected may have dark circles under the eyes and a yellowish cast, particularly around the mouth. This remedy is helpful for cold sores that occur before the monthly period or during pregnancy or menopause.
- *Dulcamara* (bittersweet) is for blisters that form in clusters and ooze watery fluid and lesions with brown crusts with reddish brown borders. Individual is prone to damp and cold and rapid changes in weather conditions.
- *Hyland's Cold Sores and Fever Blister* combination remedy (also known as Hyland's #27) made by Standard Homeopathic is formulated to alleviate the symptoms of cold sores, fever blisters, and cracked lips from acid

in food. However, you may find that an individual remedy works better, depending on your specific symptoms.

**Other homeopathic preparations for oral and genital herpes outbreaks include:** *Phosphorus* for cold sores that appear above the lip line and itch or cause sharp pain; *Petroleum* is indicated when sores develop loose crusts around the mouth, and *Apis* can be helpful for blisters around the lips that sting, itch, or burn. *Graphites* is used when the blisters emit a honey-colored fluid then crust over or have painful cracks around the mouth. *Nitric acidum* is for blisters or ulcers on the mouth, tongue, or genitals that cause sharp pain and may bleed easily. *Capsicum* is when sores burn like hot pepper, with accompanying depression or homesickness; *Tellerium* when eruptions are concurrent with back or sciatica pains), and *Thuja,* for people who have a history of warts).

**The two most common homeopathic remedies for genital herpetic eruptions** are *Natrum muriaticum* when pearl-like blisters appear and the area feels hot and swollen and *Petroleum* for symptoms are worse in the winter and better in the summer or when herpes spreads to the anus, perineum, or thighs or occurs at the onset of menstruation; sores occur in patches, appear dark red, and are tender and moist.

### Aromatherapy

Essential oils are at the heart of aromatherapy and have been used for hundreds of years to enhance well-being. Joni Loughran, author, licensed cosmetologist, and consultant to several natural cosmetics manufacturers, explains in *Natural Skin Care* (Frog Ltd., 1996) that essential oils are a concentrated form of plant energy, extracted from many parts of an aromatic plant. They are much more potent than similarly dried herbs, she says.

"Aromatherapy and the use of essential oils does not cure herpes simplex 1 (oral), herpes simplex 2 (genital), or herpes zoster (shingles), but it can relieve the symptoms, reduce pain, and shorten the length of time of sores are present," says Loughran. "Because of aromatherapy's popularity, adulterated essential oils commonly abound. When treating herpes, it's important to use high-quality, pure essential oils."

According to Loughran, essential oils with antiviral properties are most helpful against herpesvirus. The ones that have shown to be safe and effective are:

- Tea tree – has antiviral, anti-inflammatory, antiseptic, and immune boosting properties. The combination of these properties makes this oil an excellent topical treatment for herpes.
- Melissa – another excellent overall oil for herpes with powerful and gentle antiviral properties. As it may cause an allergic reaction, care should be taken to apply the oil directly on the sore. Avoid surrounding tissue. While this is an expensive oil, Loughran says it is easily found in an unadulterated form. Can be combined with rose.
- Eucalyptus – offers antiviral, anti-inflammatory, and antiseptic characteristics while reducing pain.

The following oils are good to combine with the antiviral oils mentioned above, as they reduce the discomfort associated with herpes lesions:

- Roman chamomile and German chamomile for reducing inflammation

- Bergamot (when combined with tea tree oil)
- Lavender cleanses the area while reducing pain and inflammation
- Lemon citrus oil acts as a powerful antiseptic along with stimulating immunity. *Caution: Stay out of the sun when using this oil.*

### Essential Oil Combinations

*For cold sores, fever blisters, or facial herpes (HSV-1):*

Mix together 3 drops Roman chamomile, 2 drops tea tree oil, 2 drop bergamot, and 2 drops eucalyptus. Apply to sore 3 times daily until sore begins to heal. This mixture should not be used if skin is exposed to sunlight as bergamot reacts under sunlight. Combine 3 drops of tea tree oil, 3 drops Melissa, and 4 drops of lavender. Apply 1 drop to sore, 3 times daily until sore begins to heal.

* * *

Each blend can be used as a compress by adding the ingredients to 2 cups cold water. Soak washcloth in mixture, wring out, and apply to affected area.

*For genital herpes (HSV-2):*

Mix 3 drops tea tree oil, 3 drops Melissa, 3 drops Roman chamomile, and 1 drop lavender or rose oil. Add 2 tablespoons of carrier oil (canola or sunflower oil). Apply to affected area 2-4 times daily.

* * *

As a compress: combine 3 drops Melissa, 3 drops lavender, 2 drops bergamot, and 2 drops tea tree oil with 2 cups cold water. Soak washcloth in mixture, wring out, and apply to affected area. Apply 2-4 times daily.

To maintain the integrity of these essential oil mixtures, store in brown or dark blue glass bottles with a tight cap and place in a cool, dark place.
*Note: Discontinue use if skin becomes irritated.*

## Kitchen Recipes

- ☾ Apply warm *whole* milk compresses on the lesions to help along the healing process.
- ☾ Apply a warm washcloth to the affected area several times a day. Follow with an ice pack made up of ice chips or cubes broken into small pieces wrapped in the center of a towel. Don't apply ice directly to lesion.
- ☾ Concentrated wine tannins. To obtain, set aside a small glass with a small amount of red wine and allow to sit overnight. Take a dampened cotton swab to transfer the dried wine to facial lesions.
- ☾ Bergamot (Earl Grey) tea. Place a cold, wet tea bag or compress gently on the lesion to speed healing.

## Alternative Over-the-Counter Topical Treatments

Since 2000 there has been an explosion in the number of over-the-counter (OTC) topical remedies for cold sores. Many of these products come in lip balms or small tubes of cream and feature lidocaine or benzocaine as the primary ingredient. These are substances are topical anesthetics similar to the drug Novocain, which is used in dental work.

Lidocaine and benzocaine act only as pain relievers and do not support healing or clearing up an outbreak. They can carry side effects such as blurred vision, confusion or an irregular heartbeat. People who take cholesterol lowering or sulfa-based drugs are advised to avoid these ester class drugs. Safer alternatives for relieving the pain that often accompanies cold sores are menthol and camphor.

Topical treatments mainly serve two functions: to relieve pain and speed healing. Some of the most effective ones with the most natural ingredients are *Super Lysine Plus+Cream*™ by Quantum, Enzymatic Therapy's Cold Sore Relief™ (formerly known as *Herpilyn*™); and *Erpace*™ by Dolisos. They all come packaged in small tubes, making frequent applications convenient.

*SuperLysine Plus+ Cream* ™ contains lysine in an olive oil base along with tea tree and cajeput oils together with extracts of goldenseal, echinacea flower, calendula flower, propolis plus zinc oxide, honey, gum benzoin tincture and homeopathic lithium carbonate 3X. In addition, Quantum offers two other lip preparations for cold sores and fever blisters: *LipClear*™ ointment and *LipClear Coldstick*™ containing lysine, herbs (echinacea, goldenseal, and tea tree oil), and vitamins A, D, and E in a base of a few oils. In addition, *LipClear Coldstick*™ is petroleum-free, with an added bonus of two chemical sunscreen additives that provide SPF-15 protection. The ointment version includes zinc oxide, a very effective sun block.

All of these topicals can be applied as often as needed. According to the manufacturer, these remedies are compatible with the company's other lysine-based supplements.

Cold Sore Relief ™ (*Herpilyn* ™) was popular in Germany before its import into the United States, contains a high percentage of melissa extract (lemon balm) plus allantoin. Studies have shown the product to be very safe for fine for long-term use and for use by children. The manufacturer recommends applying daily when there are frequent recurrences of cold sores and fever blisters.

*Erpace*™ comes in a base of sweet almond oil with chamomile, oregano and marjoram combined with the homeopathic Lappa major (1X) and delivered in a slim metal container with a rollerball applicator. The formula is designed to provide dry lips with moisture and to soften dry cold sores or fever blisters. It is wax- and petroleum-free. *Erpace*™ is imported from France by Dolisos.

Less convenient are oils such as vitamin E, geranium, lemon, tea tree, or eucalyptus and tinctures such as myrrh. They can be applied directly to cold sores via a cotton swab every few hours. These herbs have been found to reduce pain and promote healing. Do not apply vitamin E capsules or oil to the eye area.

There are other OTC remedies that don't meet the natural criteria that often are more readily available than the other preparations mentioned above. However, there is one remedy that contains safe ingredients and is available at nearly every drug and mass-merchandise store in the United States: *Medicated Blistex*® lip ointment is excellent for soothing and speeding the healing of cold sores and dry, cracked corners of the mouth. Its main ingredient is allantoin with camphor (0.5%) and phenol (0.5%). Camphor is considered a safe and beneficial ingredient in skin preparations and allantoin, derived from comfrey, is particularly soothing to the skin.

**Whatever ready-made topical balm you apply, be sure to apply it generously. Apply at the first sign (tingling, itching, or burning of the lip area) of an outbreak. When lesions are present, carefully work the product into the sore as much as possible,**

If your oral herpes is triggered by exposure to strong sunlight, use a lip balm than contains sunscreen with a high SPF number. To completely block ultraviolet rays, try the bright white stuff – zinc oxide– available in drugstores or pharmacy sections of supermarkets and discount chain stores. Preparations with zinc oxide also may speed healing, as zinc oxide itself is drying.

### What Doesn't Work

Over the years, these remedies have been tried and found ineffective in relieving symptoms or treating herpes lesions:

- Lasers
- Ultrasound
- Dye-light therapy with a red dye called proflavine, a light-sensitive dye that is able to penetrate the cell and the virus inside the cell. When exposed to light, the dye supposedly disrupted the viral genes so they could not reproduce and infect other cells. Once thought to be effective, it is no longer recommended for herpes treatment and is considered by many to be dangerous.
- Antibiotics – they have no effect on herpesvirus but may be used in some cases to treat secondary infections.
- Corticosteriods – creams and ointments that contain corticosteriods are used as anti-inflammatory agents do not seem to lessen the severity of herpes and are not recommended. Lesions must be kept dry with good air circulation unless they are covered by something proven to be more beneficial than dryness such as acyclovir.

### Ineffective home remedies:

- Baking soda
- Peanut butter

- Watermelon
- Tea bags
- Cornstarch
- Buttermilk
- Peppermint oil

**Ineffective store-bought remedies:**

- Campho-Phenique®
- Listerine®
- Clorox®
- Spermicidal foam
- Acetone
- Vinegar
- Toothpaste

*Chapter 4*

# Pointers on Prevention

With herpes, an ounce of prevention is worth a pound of cure, and maybe even more so for chronic sufferers. Flare-ups, despite the best efforts to prevent them, can occur when least expected. When prevention doesn't work, natural remedies come to the rescue.

The connection of mind and body to recurrent herpes outbreaks is a relatively new theory and one worthy of serious consideration by any PWH who seeks to control future herpesvirus outbreaks. The consensus between alternative and some traditional health practitioners is that stress is the #1 precipitator of recurring herpesvirus outbreaks. Emotional stress is usually cited first, but there are physical stressors that should be considered as well.

## The Stress Connection

Oscar Gillespie, Ph.D., makes the connection between herpes outbreaks and stress in *Herpes: What to Do When You Have It* (Grosset & Dunlap, 1982). He writes that herpesvirus can become the path of least resistance for the body, since a disease such as herpes can establish a pattern within the body, thus weakening normal recovery processes and the immune system's ability to fend off invaders.

Stress, whether it's good, bad or in between, is normal and a regular part of everyone's life. Too much, though, can stretch our capacity to adapt just so far before detrimental effects occur. The most common example of this is heart disease. The combination of health problems associated with this potentially life-threatening situation are revealed usually by specific physical symptoms that are aggravated by long periods of continued stress, eating foods high in salt and fat and lack of regular exercise.

Chronic stress ratchets the body's nervous and hormonal systems up to where its built-in mechanisms for adapting to and coping with stressors begin to fray and eventually break down completely. Consequently, the body's ability to deal with foreign agents or internal changes also is impaired. Without a doubt, chronic stress puts PWH at risk for more outbreaks and possibly outbreaks that take longer to heal.

## Doing Too Much

Often the stress you experience is a direct result of doing too much, whether it's multi-tasking, packing a weekend with activities after a full work week, or feeling overwhelmed by the demands and commitments of modern life. Whether it is work, working out, socializing, or volunteering to solve another's or the world's problems, any of one of us can get caught up in them to the extent that health and well being is at risk. We live in a speed-crazed world, where doing is valued of being. American culture rewards us more for moving fast rather than going along at pace more suited to our own natural rhythms.

Learning how to slow down, even when you want to, can feel like an experiment in foolishness or frustration. But recurring bouts of herpesvirus or shingles represent a clear signal to PWH that it's time to slow down the pace of your life and make your health a top priority.

Besides the stress generated in pushing ourselves past our limits, there are other stressors in life, the ones we have no control over. These, too, can impact the frequency of herpesvirus outbreaks. For example, some women will have outbreaks only at certain points during the menstrual cycle, but the particular time can vary from woman to woman. One study suggests that more women develop recurrences 5 to 12 days before the start of their next menstrual period more often than at any other time. Even though birth control pills stop the cycling hormones, they don't appear to halt or diminish outbreaks in some women of childbearing age.

Other people can become vulnerable when taking certain medications, when they have a fever, or during brief and more often prolonged exposure to strong sunlight. Others whose mouths are sensitive may find a session in the dentist's chair can provoke or intensify an outbreak. Exposure to cold, windy, or by dry weather conditions, extremely hot food, or biting or chewing lips with your teeth also can leave skin tissue open to an assault.

## The Psychological Connection

Dr. Wayne Diamond, a naturopath and psychotherapist from the Philadelphia area, has spent many years studying the skin condition of his patients. He believes that the skin is a mirror of overall health.

"My interest in herpes began," he says, "when I noticed a high number of my patients had forms of chronic viral and bacterial infections." Diamond then initiated several clinical research projects that eventually turned up a distinct connection between stress, anxiety, nutrition, and the glandular processes and how they affect the health of the skin.

According to Diamond, there are two specific emotional states that almost universally precede herpes outbreaks in those who are susceptible. One is internalizing feelings such as anger or fear (anxiety) in times of conflict, and the other is ambivalence or fear of loss. Left unacknowledged or unexpressed, can put PWH at risk for recurring infections.

He believes that these two mental conditions can effectively diminish the power of the human glandular system, which has a tremendous impact on immune function. "When people experience stress and anxiety, their bodies undergo immense changes," he says. "Body temperature increases and interferes with how nutrients are absorbed, then large amounts of acid pour into the stomach that then get absorbed into the bloodstream."

"We cannot always control when the fear of loss will arise, but we can control the resulting emotions or physical responses to it," explains Dr. Diamond. "If we can directly communicate the emotions related to fear, anger or sadness, our stress levels become greatly reduced."

Another perspective comes from author Frank Fruedberg (*Herpes: A Complete Guide to Relief and Reassurance* published in 1987 by Running Press) changing the way you think about herpes. Psychologists, he writes, often recommend to patients that they imagine the sores are a result of an allergy. "In a very real way, you are allergic to herpesvirus . . . some people are immune to them, never developing herpes simplex lesions, no matter how often they are exposed," he explains. Another way to put the situation into perspective is to think in terms of simply having cold sores, even though they below the waist.

## Reducing Anxiety and Stress

There are many ideas, books and workshops on how to cope with stress. This booklet won't attempt to give the subject detailed coverage, but, instead offer some ideas to get you thinking about getting a handle on stress so it doesn't bring on more outbreaks or prolong them.

Stress consultant and author of more than a dozen self-help books that deal with life's ups and downs, Richard Carlson, Ph.D., reminds us to "not sweat the small stuff because it's all small stuff." He finds that much of our anxiety and inner struggle stems from our busy, overactive minds always needing something to entertain them, something to focus on, always wondering what's next. Just like our bodies, he writes, our minds need an occasional break from their hectic routine. Instead of trying to raise your tolerance to stress, Carlson suggests your aim should be to lower it. Excellent advice for putting the age of (over) information, multitasking and extreme sports into perspective.

Another popular author Joan Bornysenko, Ph.D., reminds us that when our energy is tied up in useless worry and fight-or-flight, the natural tendency toward growth and wholeness is ignored or forgotten. She discovered meditation as the place where we access the relaxation response and become aware of the attitudes and thought patterns we have that produce stress. Bornysenko calls it "freeing the inner physician."

Here are some other stress-taming ideas that could work for you:

- *Learn how to say no.* This doesn't mean you say no to every offer, but to reduce the number of automatic "yeses to the ones that cut into your day and eventually take a toll on your physical and emotional health.

  Think before you say yes or no. Take the time to make the right decision for you. Offer "Let me think about it. I'll get back to you tomorrow." Agree to things that matter most to you. Another tactic that works is saying "Yes and if" at the same time. Negotiate the conditions under which you will do something.

  When only a firm "no" will do, say it with a smile. When a refusal is delivered politely and pleasantly without defense or explanation, it usually is graciously accepted. If not, don't knuckle under to manipulation. Some people will get mad, not matter what you say or do. Accept it. You'll be healthier and happier for it.

  Practice in advance if you find yourself saying "yes" too many times to requests that infer with your priorities. You'll be surprised how well this tactic works in reducing feelings of obligation to do more than you really should do.

- *Get at least 8 hours of sleep.* Preferably more if you can. Sleep serves as the physical and mental body's daily tune-up and opportunity for repair. Lack of sleep or anxiety and depression takes your body off course, leaving it open to another round of sores and discomfort. *A bedtime is 10 p.m. or earlier promotes the most healing and restful sleep and allows for the body's major organs to restore themselves.*

- *Meditate.* Substantial evidence exists that meditation supports the immune system by lowering stress, lends a genuine sense of well being and tranquility, and helps with negative states of mind as it works on the autonomic nervous system, the part of the body where the flight-or-fight mechanism resides. Start out slow: 5 minutes in the morning and evening, and add a minute each day until you are meditating for 20-30 minutes daily.

- *Exercise.* Study after study concludes 30 minutes of regular mild aerobic exercise such as walking boosts immunity and reduces stress. However, too much and too long can have the opposite effect. Pace yourself, but get out there and move.
- *Simplify and organize.* Maintaining your stuff takes time and energy and thus can be a source of stress. Best-selling author Elaine St. James, who has written three books based on her personal experience of unwinding and finding what's important to her, has discovered that there are inner and outer components to the process. The best way to do one or both is to do it slowly over time. St. James recommends one drawer, one closet, one bookshelf at a time.
- *Avoid highs-stress foods*. This includes anything that passes the moderation threshold. Go out of your way to pass on foods that contain high amounts of sugar and caffeine. Both substances can jangle your nerves and deplete the nutrients your body needs to manage stress. Adding foods high in B vitamins such as brown rice, barley, soybeans, lentils, and chickpeas can help your body cope when anxiety hits. Magnesium supplements also may help.
- Take a walk. Opt for an adult "time out" when it all becomes too much. Any kind of aerobic exercise (running, swimming, cycling) reduces tension and depression and relaxes muscles.
- Cry. The benefits of a good bawl are well documented. More than 100 years ago Charles Darwin noted the soothing effects of a good cry. Modern research indicates that tears may remove the anxiety-causing

hormone prolactin produced by the pituitary gland when we're under stress. This build-up cans actually "cried-out" of the body. Alternative practitioners often encourage their patients to cry often as it cleanses the liver, an essential body organ affected by toxins and angry feelings.

- *Listen to music.* A proven anxiety reducer, music can lower blood pressure and help stabilize heart rate.
- *Pet your pet.* Medical research proves time and again that pets are a boon to our mental and physical well-being.
- *Stop. Smile. Take a deep breath.* To keep your mind on an even keel, take a moment every half-hour or hour and stop to smile and indulge yourself in a deep breath. Visualize your worries and problems being carried away with your exhale. Deep, slow breathing automatically calms the mind and refreshes the body.
- *Read.* Considered a natural sedative by some medical experts, it's a cheap and ready escape from daily pressures.
- *Take a bath.* Water has been soothing souls and psyches for centuries. A warm to hot bath with at least 2 cups of Epsom salts can leave you feeling relaxed and refreshed.
- *Put yourself first.* Sound selfish? Not really. When demands on your time and energy climb, taking care of you almost automatically takes a back seat. To keep your defenses up against stress-related illnesses, you must eat right, get enough sleep, take regular exercise, and avoid sugar, alcohol, and cigarettes. Think of it this way: How can you be of any real use or service if you deplete your own inner resources?
- *Set boundaries.* The psychological stresses involved with having herpes, especially genitally herpes, cannot be underestimated. For many, the many emotions that come with herpes can sometimes feeling over-

whelming or impossible to overcome. Concern over what other people think about you or your condition and fear of rejection need not consume you. Trying to control the reactions or emotions of others is frustrating, exhausting and ultimately doesn't change anything. If you find it difficult to manage on your own, seek professional counseling, herpes support group or books on cognitive therapy. Highly-recommended is *Feeling Good: The New Mood* Therapy by David Burns, M.D., (Penguin Putnam, 1999) for dealing with anxiety, depression, self-defeating attitudes and habits and how to respond appropriately to others.

☾ *Do nothing.* A truly worthwhile pursuit, especially for PWH. Taking the time to disconnect from your routine and the busyness of every day life to reconnect with yourself and your inward compass. It can be truly rejuvenating, giving your mind and body a chance to turn its energies inward so it can revitalize and restore itself.

☾ *Develop and maintain a strong support network.* Ideally one that's made up of family and friends is important to maintaining well-being and an absolute necessity in times of stress. For PWH, joining a support group or seeking professional help, whether for biofeedback training or counseling to help you cope with having herpesvirus, can provide special support in coping. Check with your HMO, since a growing number of them now offer alternative treatments for stress. Also, more private insurers are more willing to cover alternative therapies.

☾ *Take time out to be still.* This is an easy and effective way to bring peace to your life by consciously removing all distractions (reading, watching TV, talking or listening to the radio) and all physical movement. Start by sitting or lying down in a quiet place where you won't be disturbed or distracted. Then, close your eyes and turn your attention inward. Focus completely on yourself; what it feels like to be you. Use your breath as a focal point without controlling or changing it. Pay close attention to any body sensations, the thoughts that pass through your mind and what it feels like to be alive right now. Keep your body as still as possible. Start with 5 minutes and gradually build to 20, then 30 to 45 minutes. By practicing mind-body awareness, you become more relaxed and centered.

## Role of Diet and Nutrition

Next to stress, diet is second most important thing that directly affects herpes outbreaks. Eliminating as well as adding certain foods can make a big difference in your overall well-being energy level and resistance to infection. Keep in mind that PWH should eat foods that help keep their bodies in balance.

Holistic herpes health care pioneer Wayne Diamond also strongly endorses a proactive dietary stance against herpesvirus. Since your skin is your first line of defense or barrier against germs, viruses, and bacteria, he says a healthy mucous membrane is probably your body's second-best defense and important to blocking the transmission of herpesvirus. To keep it healthy and strong, he says, PWH must minimize foods that promote acidity or place a strain on your digestive system, such as commercial red meat, products made from cow's milk, peanut butter, dried foods, cooked nuts, fried eggs, white flour, and gluten. Also avoid sugar, chocolate, and tomatoes, foods that often cause allergies. The vitamins important to keeping mucous membranes healthy and strong include vitamin A and beta-carotene, vitamin C with bioflavonoids, and water-soluble B vitamins.

Diamond further recommends staying away from high-acid foods, including sugar, white flour, MSG, fried foods, red meat, nightshade vegetables (tomatoes, eggplant, green peppers, and white potatoes), citrus, hard cheeses, black tea, and coffee. Dairy products and vinegar should be consumed only in small amounts.

To promote alkalinity, Diamond advocates a diet with plenty of green vegetables (but skip head lettuce as it has no nutritional value), grains, brown rice, pasta (replace red sauce with white or pesto sauce), yams, salads (garnished with a small amount of dressing), and noncitrus fruits. As proteins, fish and fowl are excellent, particularly good in colder weather. Top selections for vegetable proteins include beans, tofu, and tempeh. Avoiding foods high in the amino acid arginine — nuts, peanuts, seeds, excessive cereal grains, and chocolate. The dietary guidelines suggested by Diamond apply to all forms of herpesvirus and, he says, are equally beneficial to other chronic viral and bacterial skin conditions such as eczema, psoriasis, and acne.

Making the right food choices may be the shortest route to controlling herpesvirus outbreaks, since the kinds of foods you don't eat can make the difference in controlling herpesvirus flare-ups. However, for changes in fundamental living habits such as diet to succeed, you have to be ready and willing to make and stick to dietary changes. Look at it this way: If you're sick of being sick, then giving up the occasional treat won't seem like such a big deal. The tradeoff is exchanging a momentary pleasure for the long-term gain of missing out on the pain and suffering of a herpes flare-up. Another word for it is discipline.

## The Lysine-Arginine Connection

According to Richard S. Griffith, M.D., infectious disease specialist and professor emeritus of medicine at Indiana University School of Medicine, if you feed herpesvirus enough of the right stuff —the amino acid arginine— it may grow furiously, prodding the body to make cold sores, genital blisters, and other symptoms. The alternative is to starve the virus, subduing it so it can't cause much trouble.

The right stuff for starving herpesvirus is the amino acid lysine, which has been found over and over again in clinical and laboratory tests to suppress the growth of herpesvirus. One theory says lysine wraps a protective coat around the cell, barring the virus from penetrating and weakening the cell. Griffith believes it is the balance of power, between the two amino acids not just the amount of them that determines whether the virus takes over cells and flourishes.

The following foods have high ratios of arginine to lysine and tend to stimulate growth of the herpesvirus and should not be eaten during outbreaks, even if these foods do not trigger outbreaks.

## Foods High in Arginine

- Chocolate
- Nuts, especially peanuts, brazil nuts, cashews, hazelnuts, pecans, walnuts, almonds, and sunflower seeds
- Gelatin (Jell-O), even the kind sold in health food stores

During times of physical or emotional stress, PWH also should cut down on or eliminate these potentially troublesome foods:

- Coconut
- Popcorn
- Barley
- Corn
- Oats
- Wheat
- White bread, pasta, and rice
- Brussels sprouts
- Peas

Nuts, particularly peanuts because they are high in the amino acid arginine, have gained a infamous reputation for causing herpesvirus outbreaks in some, but not all PWH. A negative reaction to nuts is highly individual. If you're not sure nuts are a primary cause of your outbreaks, Griffith suggests experimenting by eating a small amount of peanuts, about 3 ounces or so, before going to bed. If you react, you should know the next morning.

Dr. Wayne Diamond also strongly endorses a proactive dietary stance against herpesvirus. He makes the point that since your skin is your first line of defense or barrier against germs, viruses, and bacteria, a healthy mucous membrane is probably your body's second-best defense and important to blocking the transmission of herpesvirus. To keep it healthy and strong, he says, PWH must minimize foods that promote acidity or place a strain on your digestive system. Diamond recommends staying away from high-acid foods, including sugar, white flour and similar grains, chocolate, seeds, MSG, fried foods, red meat, nightshade vegetables (tomatoes, eggplant, green peppers, and white potatoes), citrus, hard cheeses, black tea and coffee, including the decaf versions. Dairy products and vinegar should be consumed only in small amounts.

To promote alkalinity, Diamond advocates a diet with plenty of green vegetables (skip head lettuce as it has no nutritional value), grains, brown rice, pasta (replace red sauce with white or pesto sauce), yams, salads (garnished with a small amount of dressing), and noncitrus fruits. For protein, fish and fowl are excellent and particularly good for the body in colder weather. Top selections for vegetable proteins include beans, tofu, and tempeh. The dietary guidelines suggested by Diamond apply to all forms of herpesvirus and are equally beneficial to other chronic viral and bacterial skin conditions such as eczema, psoriasis and acne.

## Acid-Producing Foods to Avoid

Foods that increase internal acidity seem to encourage the activating herpesvirus. The virus loves acidity, growing three times faster in this environment. In general, if the body produces excess acid that can't be neutralized or eliminated by the liver, lungs and kidneys, illnesses, a herpes outbreak, can occur. A build-up of acid in the body results in inflammation and pain. Individuals differ on how much and how well their body metabolizes and rids itself of excess acid.

### *Foods to Avoid*

- Coffee (including decaf), black tea, cocoa
- White bread and baked goods (pastries, cookies, bagels, muffins, scones, and croissants)

- Cow's milk, yogurt and cheese
- Products made with wheat flour (bread, cakes, pastries, cereals)
- Citrus fruits
- Fried foods
- Spicy foods
- Red meat (beef, lamb, pork)
- Pizza
- Chocolate
- Dry-roasted nuts (especially almonds, brazil nuts, cashews, hazelnuts, peanuts, pecans and walnuts), potato chips and salty snack foods
- Anything with high fructose corn syrup or sugar
- Processed lunch meats, spreads, and processed cheese
- Conventionally made jellies and jams
- Soft drinks
- Alcohol (beer, wine, spirits)
- Ketchup and mayonnaise
- Black pepper, excessive salt, mustard
- White vinegar
- Baking soda
- Aluminum-based baking powder

### *Foods that Promote Acid-Alkaline Balance*

- All vegetables (especially kale and broccoli) and herbs
- Fruits (except citrus) and dried fruit (in moderation because of high sugar content)
- Legumes (lentils, chickpeas, kidney beans)
- Whole grains, especially millet. White rice (jasmine, basmati) is okay because it's easy to digest. Also oats, 100% rye crispbread and sugar-free granola.

- Fish
- Goat milk products including yogurt and cheese
- Vegetable oils
- Carob and molasses
- Herbal tea, grain coffee
- Unsweetened fruit juices
- Nuts and seeds (particularly pine nuts, pumpkin seeds and sunflower seeds) in moderation
- Miso soup

*Foods to Eat Sparingly (twice a week at most)*

- Eggs
- Poultry
- Tomatoes
- Butter
- Smoked or canned fish

## The Sugar Trap

Sugar is like sunshine: a little can boost your energy and spirits, but too much can be harmful.

Besides tasting good, it also causes the brain to release feel-good chemicals such as serotonin and endorphins. While most of us are born with the instinct to seek out the sweet stuff, too often we develop cravings for sugar that follow us into adulthood. Heavy sugar consumption has been linked to premature aging, several degenerative diseases, cardiovascular disease, liver dysfunction, type II diabetes, osteoporosis, gum disease, weight gain and impaired immunity. Sugar can weaken the gastrointestinal tract and interfere with food digestion and assimilation. A healthy digestive system is crucial to good immune function. This is important to all of us, but particularly to PWH, because maintaining a healthy immune system is key to keeping herpesvirus in check.

Author and well-known nutritionist Ann Louise Gittleman calls sweet foods "a devil in disguise." In her book *Get the Sugar Out: 501 Simple Ways to Cut the Sugar Out of Any Diet* (Crown Trade Paperbacks, 1996), Gittleman takes a realistic look at the effects of sugar on the body and offer tips and recipes to eliminate sugar from any type of diet. She and other experts agree that refined sugar acts more like a drug that our bodies need to detoxify than a nutrient-supplying food . . . our bodies have to use their own mineral reserves just to digest it.

Sugar stalls the immune system by 1) preventing white blood cells from doing their job as germ killers; 2) reducing the body's ability to produce antibodies (the proteins that combine with and deactivate foreign invaders such as viruses); 3) hindering the transport of vitamin C, a nutrient crucial to overall immune function; 4) upsetting the balance of crucial minerals such as magnesium and calcium; and 5) neutralizing the effects of essential fatty acids and allowing cells to be more open to invasion by allergens and microorganisms.

Medical studies have found that the immune system's antibody production drops off after as little as 18 grams of sugar — about as much as in a half-can of soda. Sugar also interferes with the way the body absorbs B vitamins that are crucial to keeping herpesvirus in check and maintaining a healthy nervous system. The ideal way for the body to ingest sugar properly is through eating whole foods, especially complex carbohydrates that allow for gradual introduction of sugars into the bloodstream.

The key here is to satisfy your sweet tooth without risking your health. Blood sugar equilibrium, Gittleman says, is one of the most important but overlooked keys to health.

Here are some guidelines to follow:

- Eat foods that rank between zero and 40 on the Glycemic Index. Foods such as sweet potatoes, slow-cooked oatmeal, grapes (in moderation), apples, mangos, pears, lentils, yogurt and soybean bring blood sugar up gradually and contribute to its stability. If you eat foods that fall in the moderate or high glycemic levels (such as potatoes, carrots, applesauce, corn chips, most commercial cold breakfast cereals), eat them with a helping of protein to help slow down the body's insulin response. (Check ratings for individual foods at www.glycemicindex.com)
- Replace refined sugars with natural sugars such as stevia, pure maple syrup, barely malt, rice syrup or pureed fresh fruit. Avoid honey and fructose – especially high fructose corn syrup, found, unfortunately, in most processed foods. Not only is it blamed for the increased rates of obesity, high fructose corn syrup is hard for the body to digest. Personally, I have found stevia, in moderate amounts, to be very satisfying and compatible with my metabolism. Still, it is important to use natural replacement sugars sparingly. There's no fooling the body!
- Read food labels religiously for the number of sugar grams for *each serving*. The Nutrition Facts box printed on nearly all food products lists a product's sugar contact near the bottom of the carbohydrates section. Select foods that contain 5 to 7 grams or less of sugar per serving.
- Aim to keep daily sugar consumption under 40 grams, and between 20 and 40 grams if you have regular herpesvirus recurrences. A teaspoon of refined white sugar contains 4 grams of sugar.

- If you crave sugar, try eating 4 to 6 small meals that contain some quality protein. This will give your blood sugar a fighting chance to even out and you should eventually find sweets less tempting. Often, sugar cravings can become more manageable by adding more protein to your diet. Be sure to stay away from fat-free foods. Besides being highly processed, they contain even more sugar than the higher fat version of the same food to make up for the lack of fat. Also, avoid foods high in carbohydrates such as bread, bagels, and pasta that are high in simple sugars and contribute to spikes in blood sugar.
- Substitute complex carbohydrates for simple ones, as the complex variety requires longer digestion to be absorbed. Foods especially beneficial for PWH include legumes (lentils, chickpeas, kidney beans) and vegetables such a yams, broccoli, and zucchini. These foods with long sugar chains, like complex carbohydrates, release their sugars into the bloodstream gradually and supply the body with a more consistent, even flow of energy. Consider starting your day with a bowl of slow-cooked oats. Slow-cooked oats have been shown to help regulate blood sugar and have a positive effect on the nervous system.
- To keep blood sugar constant, aim for a diet that is approximately 40 percent carbohydrates, 30 percent protein and 30 percent fat.
- Go through your pantry and cupboards and toss out candy, cookies, sugary cereals, conventional white bread and pasta. Throw it or give it all away and promise not to replace it. If you must have the food, make a special trip for it and buy only a small quantity.
- Spike foods with cinnamon. It helps balance blood sugar by raising insulin, according to studies conducted at the U.S. Department of Agriculture.

- For safe and satisfying dessert, mix up a batch of raw almonds (soaked in water overnight or for 2 to 3 hours minimum), sprinkle 1 or 2 teaspoons of plain cocoa powder over them, then mix thoroughly with a tablespoon of barely malt syrup and enjoy.
- Enlist the aid of supplements. Regular intake of glucose tolerance factor (GTF) version of chromium is recommended over chromium picolante to stabilize blood sugar, particularly if you have been a heavy consumer of sweets, bread and pasta. Take 200-600 mcg daily. For strong or overwhelming sugar cravings, Ann Louise Gittleman recommends taking 500 mg of the amino acid l-glutamine 2 to 3 times daily. The brain converts l-glutamine to glutamic acid, the only source of glucose besides sugar the brain uses for energy.
- The antioxidant alpha lipoic acid has shown promise in helping diabetics control their blood sugar. About 50 mg a day should help curb cravings. In addition, be sure you're getting enough magnesium, at least 300-500 mg daily; increase intake if cravings (particularly for chocolate) are stronger before menstruation. Other vitamins and minerals important to maintaining blood sugar balance are zinc, manganese, B complex, vitamin C, and pantothenic acid.
- Eleutherococcus (formerly called Siberian ginseng) also curbs sugar cravings, and keeps energy levels steady while nourishing the adrenal glands.

If stress triggers sugar binges, you also should take formulas specifically to support adrenal and pancreas functions. Stress and sugar represent a harmful combination to the adrenal glands, that help your body cope with stress. The adrenal glands are closely associated with function of the kidney and liver. These two vital body organs that rely on proper nutrition and adequate rest for functioning.

Sugar has been proven to block the absorption or speed up the elimination of B vitamins and nearly all minerals. After you eat sugar, both calcium and magnesium are eliminated from the body when you urinate. According to Gittleman, no matter how much of these minerals you take in food or supplemental form, if you take them with a lot of sugar, you will not be able to absorb them.

Balanced blood sugar is the result of consuming sufficient protein and essential fatty acids. While diet experts constantly wrn about fat consumption, eating less sugar is more important to maintaining good health than eating moderate amounts of fat.

# The Slow but Sure Path to Conquering Sugar Cravings

Some people can stop an addiction cold turkey, but many of us need a more to take a more gradual approach in releasing habits that damage our health and well-being.

Banning sweets from your diet may work in the short run, but isn't practical. Here's a more middle-of-the road approach that will help lessen dependence on sugar. The following timeframes are only suggested. Take as much time as you need to complete the process of eliminating candy and sweets from your diet.

First, eliminate all *refined* sugars (this includes all artificial sweeteners such as aspartame, sucralose, Splenda plus white and brown sugar, corn syrup and high fructose corn syrup) from your diet.

For the next 1 to 4 weeks, satisfy your sweet tooth with honey, maple syrup, stevia, fruit-based sweeteners, dried fruit and small amounts of fruit juices.

Then, substitute foods made with processed sugar with fresh and dried fruits and fruit juices. Use natural sweeteners listed above sparingly. Do this for another 1 to 4 weeks.

At the three-month mark at the latest, taper off simple sugars completely except for small amounts of barley malt syrup, brown rice syrup or stevia. Eat only seasonal fresh fruit, small amounts of diluted fruit juices and dried fruits that have been soaked in water overnight.

Finally, remove all sugars from your diet except for fresh fruit in season. Concentrate on eating apples, bananas and pears since they are available year round. All are delicious when baked and pears are easily poached.

You may find that only after a couple of weeks, your desire for sugar is significantly less. By substituting fresh fruits and routinely eating whole foods, you likely will discover that treats you once found so delicious now taste cloyingly sweet or artificial. More importantly, it is possible to live your life happily, healthily and contentedly without sweets!

## Foods to Add to Your Diet

The healing components of food are becoming better understood and known every day. Ruth Winter, author of *A Consumer's Guide to Medicines in Food* (Crown Trade Paperbacks, 1995), notes the immune system is very much influenced by what we eat.

As food science makes strides in research, strange and fancy words such as *nutraceuticals* and *phytochemicals* are being bandied about. Both help in the prevention and treatment of illness and diseases. Phytochemicals is an umbrella term applied to the array of natural chemical compounds found by the thousands in such whole foods as fruits, vegetables, grains, and legumes. The magazine reported that phytochemicals are substances that give other virus- and cold-fighting vitamins in whole foods a supercharged boost.

Phytochemicals contain some important components, such as:

- *Sulforaphane:* a tumor-blocking substance found in broccoli, cauliflower, brussels sprouts, and kale.
- *Allyic Sulfides:* found in garlic and onions. These validate the claim that garlic is an excellent natural preventative for colds, flu, other infectious diseases, and chronic conditions such as stomach cancer.
- *Flavonoids* (or bioflavonoids): found in green plants, citrus fruits, and berries such as currants. These exponentially boost vitamin C absorption in the body, thereby fortifying the immune system against viruses. They also are though to block cancer-causing hormones from latching onto a cell.

### Garlic

This versatile, talented member of the onion family acts like a broad-spectrum antibiotic, killing bacteria, fungus, yeasts, viruses, and parasites and helps to eliminate toxins in the body. Hippocrates, who gave herpes its modern name, used garlic to treat infected wounds and upper respiratory infections.

To many people's dismay, conventional antibiotics don't cure viral infections. Garlic or its constituents, notes writer Paul Berner (*The Healing Power of Garlic,* Prima Press, 1996), will directly kill a variety of viruses including flu, herpes, and cytomegalovirus (CMV). It also stimulates the body's natural defenses against these invaders.

Raw garlic holds more benefit than taking it in pill form, and the purple-skinned variety is considered to possess the most medicinal properties. To get the full benefit of allicin, garlic's most active medicinal property, it must be fresh and either chopped or crushed. For best results, eat 2 to 3 raw garlic cloves daily or use that amount or more in cooking. The best way to extract allicin from garlic, Berner suggests, is to soak the garlic pieces in a mixture of water and alcohol (try a dry red wine) at room temperature for 3 hours.

Since garlic is a strong herb, side effects are possible, particularly in high doses. Two to three or more bulbs daily can cause stomach and skin irritation, nausea, diarrhea, intestinal gas, headaches, flushed skin, increased sexual desire, and insomnia. Cutting back should reduce symptoms. Any serious harm to the body by eating large quantities of garlic usually doesn't usually occur because the discomfort experienced puts the brakes on eating too much of it.

If taking garlic raw is inconvenient or too strong, try Japanese-produced Kyolic brand garlic in liquid or capsule form. While it is a less irritating form of garlic, it doesn't have as many of the benefits that raw garlic offers, but research finds there is merit in taking it, particularly as a tonic.

## Foods that Act as Medicine

Some other foods that have been shown to have antiviral and antibacterial activity, including herpes, cold, and flu viruses, include:

- Green tea — packs a high antioxidant punch
- Quinoa — a high-protein, gluten-free grain that's rich in lysine and vitamins B and C.
- Garlic — excellent, all-around helper for PWH.
- Olive leaf extract — curtails growth of viruses and bacteria. Also shown to help heal herpesvirus lesions.

## Diet Pointers

- Go out of your way to eat fresh, organic foods.
- Vary your diet. Try to eat different foods every day.
- Begin every day with a healthy breakfast. Anything goes for breakfast, even fish and veggies.
- Avoid hydrogenated oils, food additives, artificial colors, preservatives, stabilizers, and chemicals such as nitrates BHA and BHT.
- Eat processed foods sparingly; Especially commercially prepared ice creams, sodas (colas in particular), and candies especially fall into this category.
- Stay away from refined carbohydrates and refined sugar. The body must draw on its reserves to break down sugar while using up its supplies of vitamins $B_1$, $B_2$, $B_6$, niacin, magnesium, and others. *Eating sugar and other highly processed sweeteners (especially corn syrup and high fructose corn syrup) weakens the blood and lowers immune function.* Also, eating a diet heavy on grains,

whole or not, can upset the body's balance and set the stage for an outbreak.

- Focus on eating quality proteins. Foods that contain all of the essential 8 amino acids are called first-class proteins, and are found in animal, vegetable, dairy, and seafood products. Your body's requirements for protein depend on the overall condition of your health, current stress level and how well you synthesize the protein you consume. Vary the amounts and kinds of proteins you eat for maximum assimilation. If you are economically and ecologically inclined, mix grains and legumes and to meet the body's need for protein.
- Juicing is one of the best ways to get your vegetables and increase your intake of beta-carotene and zinc. Especially beneficial to PWH are combinations of beets, carrots, celery, and parsley juices, as they are natural liver cleansers. Add fresh apple, garlic, or ginger for variety.
- The Chinese have used shiitake mushrooms for centuries to foster resistance to infection. A compound called lentinan found in the mushrooms has been found to increase immune function by stimulating interferon and T-cell production. Shiitake mushrooms are available in fresh and dry forms and make an excellent side dish.
- Try eating edible seaweed. In experiments conducted in the 1970s on the effect of different kinds of seaweed from the red marine algae family on HSV-1 and HSV-2, spread of virus was reduced by 50 percent and diminished the viability of the pro-herpes activity by 100 percent. One species in particular, Cryptosiphonia woodii, a microalgae found in the inner-tidal pools scattered along the Pacific coast, was found by Scripps Institute to hold back herpesvirus.

- Eat only when hungry and only until hunger subsides. Push away the plate when you are about two-thirds full.
- Chew your food slowly and completely.
- Pause and be grateful for what you already have.

**Both clinical research and anecdotal evidence have shown repeatedly that diet is the most effective in preventing recurrences of herpes outbreaks or in thwarting herpesvirus symptoms in their initial stages**

# Homemade Yogurt Recipe

Yogurt contains essential good bacteria that are helpful to the digestive and respiratory tracts and the immune system.

When made *without* refined sweeteners such as sugar and high fructose corn syrup, it is an especially beneficial food for PWH. Since many commercial yogurts contain sweeteners that prompt adverse reaction in PWH, making your own provides an easy and thrifty solution to store-bought brands.

For the most healthful yogurt, start with organic cow's or goat's milk and plain yogurt with *live cultures* or a packet of powdered yogurt culture.

To make the first batch, you'll most likely use store-bought yogurt as a starter. A brand with live cultures is essential since the other kind won't work as a starter. For variety, you can use single-flavored yogurts such as lemon or vanilla.

Select a good-size glass jar (16 oz.- 32 oz.) with a screw-top lid. Fill the jar with milk, leaving about 1/2-inch to 1-inch of room at the top. Pour the measured milk into a saucepan. Heat milk over medium or low heat until it reaches 185°. (A simple clip-on glass candy thermometer works great.) Be sure to keep an eye on the heating milk as it can easily boil over.

Turn off the heat and remove the milk from the stove. Let milk cool until it reaches about 110°. Mix or whisk in about 2 tablespoons of starter yogurt. Pour mixture back into the jar and place lid on tightly. Then wrap the jar in a kitchen towel and hold in place with a rubber band. Place wrapped jar on a heating pad set to low or over the pilot light on a gas stove, and cover jar with a large pot or mixing bowl for 24 hours.

The key to making yogurt "set" is a correct, constant temperature. If the temperature is too warm, the live bacteria in the culture die.

Homemade yogurt lasts about 5 days in the refrigerator before turning too tart. Understand the homemade version is often is not as thick or creamy as the store-bought variety.

## Vitamins, Minerals, Amino Acids, and Herbs

Earl Mindell, R.Ph., Ph.D., author of the *Vitamin Bible* (Warner Books, 1985), defines vitamins as organic substances necessary for life in all its forms – growth, metabolism, and physical and mental health. Vitamins are essential to the normal functioning of our bodies and, with few exceptions, cannot be synthesized or manufactured by our bodies. In their natural state, they are found in minute quantities in all organic food, so to head off deficiencies or to supplement what our diets don't normally supply, it's particularly important for PWH to take supplements. There are 13 organic substances called vitamins and 18-plus chemicals known as minerals and 8 amino acids that have been identified for proper body function and maintaining good health. Different vitamins, however, fulfill different needs. Some aid the work of enzymes and others join up with hormones that affect the glands and subsequently other organs. Others have a definite role in cellular and immune functions.

The established allowances for vitamins and minerals set by the U.S. government through the Recommended Dietary Allowance (RDA) are automatically low since they are set to meet the *minimum* amount of a vitamin and mineral required to avoid gross nutritional deficiencies. In fact, Roger Williams, Ph.D., who discovered pantothenic acid some 40 years ago, also suggested the idea of "biochemical individuality." He maintains that while we all need the same nutrients, the amount can differ greatly from person to person.

Janet Zand, N.D., O.M.D., L.Ac., and co-founder of McZand Herbal, believes that the fruits and vegetables grown today lack the nutritional punch of produce grown earlier in this century. Overworked, chemically treated soils and pollutants have resulted in a food supply deficient in the vitamins and minerals necessary to defend against serious and chronic illnesses, she says. Zand also favors tailoring supplement intake and dosage to daily or seasonal need and varying manufacturers of the most frequently taken supplements.

While there is no consensus on how large dosages should be for PWH to maintain health, some practitioners have made recommendations. You should, though, experiment to determine what's best for your particular health situation. Some supplements such as vitamin A should not be taken in excess. Please read labels carefully and consult with the appropriate healthcare professional when in doubt.

In a report issued in July 1996 by the *Council for Responsible Nutrition News*, the National Institutes of Health said that physically active adults many need increased amounts of some vitamins including $B_1$ (thiamin), $B_2$ (riboflavin), and $B_6$ (pyridoxine). Exercise is believed to burn up more of these three nutrients. These B vitamins are involved in the metabolic reactions that produce energy. In the same report, the antioxidants vitamin C, E, beta-carotene and selenium were found to be important in repairing the oxidative damage caused by the release of free radicals during exercise. Stress and air pollution also tax our bodies' resources, and when ill from a viral or bacterial invasion, the body uses up more vitamins and minerals than normal.

**The vitamins and minerals that support a strong, responsive immune system are A, E, C, $B_6$, selenium, and zinc.**

**Vitamin A** – important antioxidant and crucial to immune function, manufactures red blood cells and supports health of skin, mucous membranes, hair, and eyes. Also necessary for producing lysozyme, an antibacterial enzyme found in sweat, tears and saliva. (15,000-25,000 I.U.) *Sources:* all yellow fruits and green vegetables, especially in apricots, beets, carrots, alfalfa, egg yolk, broccoli, dairy products and fish oils.

**Beta-carotene** – is a precursor to vitamin A and converts into the vitamin as the body needs it. Although vitamin A can cause toxicity when high dosages are consumed, beta-carotene has no such restrictions, as the body uses only what it needs. It also increases the action of interferon, which the body uses to stop viruses from multiplying, and the action of white blood cells against viruses. In addition, research done in Germany indicates beta-carotene may protect the skin against UV exposure. (10,000-15,000 I.U.) Sources: orange and yellow fruits and vegetables.

**B complex** – as a group, these vitamins protect against disease and infections by supporting immune function. Also useful in repairing tissue, strengthening mucous membrane, helping to build blood, and buffering the body against the effects of stress. Helps the body use sugars, fats, and proteins. Recommended dosage is in a complex formula, as it often works with other nutrients as it increases the production of hydrochloric acid, which is necessary for digestion. (50-100 mg 1-3 times daily). *Sources:* most fruits and vegetables; particularly brewer's yeast, whole grains, liver, and kidney.

In addition to B complex, individual B vitamins, such as $B_5$ and $B_6$ can be taken as needed for specific support while under stress.

☾ *$B_1$ (thiamin):* aids in converting carbohydrates into energy; necessary for a healthy nervous system, good vision, skin, hair, and nails. *Sources:* fortified cereals, meats, slow cooked oatmeal, and split peas.

☾ *$B_2$ (riboflavin):* helps metabolize protein, sugar, fats, and lipids into energy; supplies oxygen to cells; important for red blood cell growth; used by skin and nails. Easily depleted when under stress. *Sources:* milk, cottage cheese, egg whites, brewer's yeast, broccoli, lamb, chicken, beef, and bread.

☾ *$B_3$ (niacin):* essential to mental and emotional health; releases energy and stimulates circulation; delivers histamines to the bloodstream; metabolizes food into energy; important for maintaining healthy skin. Reduces tension, fatigue, and insomnia. *Sources:* poultry, lean meat, fish, and peanuts.

☾ *$B_5$ (pantothenic acid):* important for metabolizing food and producing essential body chemicals; supports formation of antibodies, stimulates adrenal function, maintains digestive tract, and protects against respiratory infections. *Sources:* organ meats, brewer's yeast, bran, sesame seeds, eggs, and soybean.

☾ *$B_6$ (pyridoxine):* helps synthesize DNA and RNA; used to produce hormones, antibodies, and red blood cells; also aids in the metabolism of fat, protein, and carbohydrates. The body's need for this vitamin is directly connected to protein intake: the more protein consumed, the more $B_6$ the body needs. *Sources:* bananas, chicken, potatoes, peas, spinach, walnuts, liver, oatmeal, and wheat germ.

☾ *$B_{12}$:* essential for normal function of all body cells, including brain and nerve cells; increases resistance to infection and is key to formation of red blood cells. *Sources:* clams, oysters, mackerel, sardines, crabs, herring, fish, muscle meats, and dairy products.

- ☾ *Biotin:* regulates function of skin, nerves, bone marrow, and reproductive glands; also helps metabolize carbohydrates and protein, folic acid, pantothenic acid, and niacin. *Sources:* egg yolks, liver, brown rice, chicken, brewer's yeast and whole-grain cereals.
- ☾ *Choline:* essential to liver function and supports the health of the myelin sheath (nerve covering); and aids in utilization of fat and cholesterol. *Sources:* Whole grains, egg yolks, legumes, cauliflower, lettuce and soy.
- ☾ *Folic acid:* central to normal cell growth, production of new red blood cells, and protein metabolism; important to immune function; synthesizes DNA and RNA. *Sources:* liver, brewer's yeast, green leafy vegetables, lentils and black-eyed peas.
- ☾ *Inositol:* nourishes the brain; reduces fat in liver. *Sources:* citrus fruits, whole grains, legumes, nuts, and seeds.

**Vitamin C (ascorbic acid)** — a natural antiviral agent that stimulates the immune system to produce interferon and enhances function of white blood cells; assists body in processing essential fatty acids (EFAs). May increase resistance to infection by activating the formation of collagen in the skin and the lining in the body's openings. Also promotes wound healing, strengthens blood vessels and helps the body to absorb iron. (3,000-6,000 mg daily or to bowel tolerance) *Sources:* most fresh fruits and vegetables; especially citrus fruits, rose hips, black currants, and peppers.

**Vitamin D** — general immunity enhancer and aid to healthy skin; important for bones, teeth, body tissue, and cartilage; and valuable to nervous system and heart; aids in blood clotting. *(200 I.U.) Sources:* eggs, milk, fish oils, and sunshine.

**Vitamin E** — greatly influences cellular immunity and helps prolong the life of red blood cells; also its antioxidant function may help in the production of antibodies. (400-800 I.U.) *Sources:* oils, almonds, sunflower seeds, whole wheat, wheat germ, peaches and prunes.

**Minerals and Trace Minerals** — important to sustaining health; works with enzymes that are important to cellular function. Deficiencies lead to increased susceptibility to infectious diseases. *Sources:* whole foods, including dairy products, fish, red meats, fruits, and vegetables.

**Calcium** — helps build bones and keep them strong and supports healthy cell membranes. *Sources:* milk, cheese, yogurt, tofu, sardines, oysters, dried apricots, broccoli, dry beans, whole-wheat bread and fortified cereals.

**Copper** — helps metabolize vitamin C and iron and promotes energy through aiding in production of prostaglandins; necessary to maintain blood, bones, skin, and circulatory system. *Sources:* liver, whole grains, seafood, almonds, and dried legumes.

**Iron** — important to immune function. Deficiency can lead to impaired white blood cell response. *Sources:* beans, peas, whole wheat, prunes, leafy green vegetables, liver and seafood.

**Magnesium** — helps transmit nerve impulses to muscles; vital in assimilation of EFAs. *Sources:* almonds and sunflower and sesame seeds.

**Manganese** — provides essential support to nervous system function and active player in resisting autoimmune illnesses. Activates enzymes necessary to release energy.

*Sources:* tropical fruits, nuts, cereals, egg yolk, and some spices (cardamom, cloves, ginger, and turmeric).

**Molybdenum** — aids in processing carbohydrates and fats and effective against mercury.
*Sources:* dark leafy green vegetables, whole grains, and legumes.

**Phosphorus** — can reduce the effects of stress. *Sources:* eggs, fish, grains, meat, poultry, cheese, legumes and milk.

**Selenium** — aids in assimilation of vitamin E and boosts the antioxidant properties already the domain of vitamin E. Plays an important role in maintaining immunity. Not much is needed by the body, but people with autoimmune diseases have been found to have consistently lower levels of selenium. *Sources:* fish, kidney, and liver; lesser sources include cereals, poultry, mushrooms, garlic, and asparagus. Dosages between 50 mg and 200 mg daily are considered safe.

**Tyrosine** — amino acid that helps the body deal with emotion stress by balancing the nervous system and preventing skin eruptions. Take 500mg twice daily on an empty stomach.

**Zinc** — considered the mineral equivalent of vitamin C and probably the most important mineral for maintaining the body's antiviral capabilities. Aids in formation of enzymes; this mineral plays a key role in the body's assimilation of vitamins, particularly B vitamins. It has been found that zinc, when taken with vitamin C, it is more effective than taking vitamin C alone. Zinc is vital for wound healing and maintaining healthy skin. However, taking too much zinc (100 mg taken for 30 days or more) can have the opposite effect on the immune system, depressing it instead of heightening its function. Continued overdosing can lead to heart, cholesterol, and thyroid problems. Its effectiveness is lessened if taken with high fiber foods, iodine, and such drugs as tetracycline, cortisone, and diuretics.

Vegetarians in particular should take zinc supplements because of their typically high-fiber diets and because the amount of phytic acid found in plant foods interferes with absorption. Zinc also competes with copper for absorption, so it's best to take both. *Sources:* oysters, meat, chicken, lean beef, milk, eggs, fish, pumpkin seeds, lima beans, oatmeal, wheat germ, sesame seeds, and brewer's yeast.

**Zinc Lozenges (zinc gluconate)** — absorbed quickly by the bloodstream; stimulates immune function to fend off viruses once they take hold in the body, or in the case of herpes, reactivated. (One lozenge daily; one every 3 to 4 hours during first sign or first 3 days of an outbreak.) ***Note: Do not take zinc tablets or capsules and zinc lozenges* at the same time.**

## Essential Supplements for PWH

- ☾ *Lysine* — to prevent the herpesvirus from replicating. Take 500 mg daily for maintenance; during an outbreak, take 500 mg, on an empty stomach, 3 to 5 times daily until lesions heal.
- ☾ *Vitamin C* — high doses of vitamin C with bioflavonoids or Ester C (vitamin C bound with calcium carbonate) should be taken when the first prodrome surfaces. Take 1,000 mg initially, followed by 500 mg, 3 to 4 times daily until you are symptom free.
- ☾ *Echinacea & Goldenseal* combination — tinctures recommended over capsules; follow directions on label. Not for long-term use. Follow package directions.

- ☾ *Garlic* – at earliest sign of an outbreak take large doses of fresh, chopped garlic with food or 12 small pills then 3 pills every 4 hours until symptoms subside.
- ☾ *Licorice root* — for immune system and adrenal gland support. Take 30 to 40 drops of tincture, 2 times daily.
- ☾ *B-complex* –– for energy and nervous system support. 50-100 mg, 3 times daily. Take with food. Extra supplementation with 50 mg $B_6$ once a day during outbreaks is advised.
- ☾ *Zinc citrate or zinc picolante*– for fighting infection. Up to 30mg daily.

## Most Beneficial Types of Exercise

While regular, mild aerobic exercise such as walking often has been proven to be an effective way to strengthen the immune system, hatha yoga takes this process a pleasant step further. By its very nature, hatha yoga is the best example of therapeutic exercise. Certified Iyengar yoga teacher, physician and author Mary Pullig Schatz explains, "Yoga postures are one way of reinforcing the message that all is well, and that normal immune function is appropriate. The body thinks 'I am being so well-fed, well-exercised, and well-rested. Let me be well.'"

Hatha yoga is especially useful in offsetting the effects of stress. Since chronic stress has a powerfully negative effect on the immune system, hatha yoga, when practiced regularly, helps the body rest and repair itself.

While there are many forms of yoga now taught, Iyengar yoga is considered the most therapeutic form of hatha yoga. It emphasizes proper alignment, uses props when necessary and makes liberal use of restorative poses. Restorative poses are done on the floor with the body supported by props in strategic places such as legs, back, arms and shoulders. This collection of yoga poses allows the both the body, mind and nervous system to rest and restore itself. They are highly recommended for PWH who have chronic outbreaks.

Other helpful types of yoga for PWH are Kripalu and Anusara yoga. PWH should steer clear of more aerobic forms of yoga such as ashtanga, power, Kundalini, Bikram or "hot" yoga until their immune systems are stronger.

Qigong (chee-gung) is a low-impact, low-stress form of exercise that offers healing benefits to PWH by cultivating, purifying and storing energy. Tested scientifically, the healing form of qigong is known to reduce stress, build stamina, enhance immunity and increase vitality and improves the function of the digestive, circulatory, respiratory, cardiovascular and lymphatic systems.

The founding form of Tai Chi, qigong is an ancient discipline that uses a combination of gentle body movements, self-applied massage, breath practice and meditation. Qigong can be practiced standing, sitting or lying down and requires no special equipment. Most of the movements are simple, require little effort to learn and fit easily into a daily routine.

The most important aspect of qigong is the exercises support the innate, powerful ability the body has to heal itself by removing blocked energy. When practiced regularly and with attention, qigong has been proven to have a profound affect on physical and mental health.

And like yoga, qigong supports and sustains the mind-body-spirit connection. An excellent resource for basic qigong exercises, breathing, relaxation and self-massage techniques can be found at *www.healerwithin.com/practice.htm.*

## Good Hygiene

Last, but certainly not least, is practicing good health habits to avoid spreading the virus.

Laboratory studies have shown that herpesvirus is sturdy virus. In 1982, UCLA researchers found that herpesvirus can live on a toilet seat for up to 4 hours, on a medical instrument for up to 18 hours and for as long as 72 hours on gauze. Because herpesvirus is so resilient, diligent adherence to good hygiene habits is one very effective way to control its spread.

While confronted with an active herpesvirus infection, PWH should be especially careful to avoid physical contact with others as well as being equally diligent with themselves. This is important since herpesvirus can be transferred to other body parts by touching an active blister and inadvertently moving active virus particles that take root somewhere else on their bodies, resulting in a new infection with its own independent pattern of recurrence frequency, duration, and severity. To avoid this, during an outbreak, wash your hands as soon as you get up, since touching sores while asleep is common.

To minimize the risk of infection to yourself and others, wash your hands — often and thoroughly with *hot* water and soap — especially after using public facilities and having contact with doorknobs, public telephones, shopping carts, facial tissues, and hand towels used by others.

Avoid sharing towels, toothbrushes, clothing, and eating utensils during an outbreak, and watch where you apply that lip balm or lipstick — keep it away from any sores so you don't infect an otherwise unaffected part of your lip.

At the first sign of infection and if blisters develop, toss your toothbrush and replace it with a fresh one and try to keep your toothbrush from touching the edge of the toothpaste tube so you don't keep spreading the virus and end up with multiple lesions. After brushing, soak your toothbrush in baking soda to fight germs and then store your toothbrush upright in a dry place. The bathroom's moist air creates an ideal breeding ground for herpesvirus.

Good hygiene also can help avoid cross-infection. If you and your partner both have HSV-1, HSV-2, or both, don't make the mistake of thinking you are immune from passing virus particles back and forth to each other during an active period. Since you both may carry a different strain of herpesvirus, it is important that you take precautions or avoid physical contact when you're contagious.

Chapter 5

# Related and Not-So Related Conditions

### *Shingles*

Herpes varicella zoster virus (HVZ), commonly known as chickenpox, is the precursor to shingles, an unpredictable and painful condition that occurs most often after age 40.

Chickenpox is transmitted by an airborne virus rather than through one-on-one contact like HSV1 and HSV2. It is estimated that 75 percent of U.S. children have the illness by age 15. Doctors considered it a viral infection of the nerve and not a skin disease. The name comes from the Latin word *singulum,* or belt, because the rash most often appears near the waist. Like HSV-1, shingles can sometimes involve the eye area, creating a condition known as herpes zoster ophthalmicus.

The virus returns when the immune system is undermined by age, disease or severe stress. Outbreaks are quite common among the elderly, who can experience more severe symptoms and longer outbreaks.

The dormant HVZ virus resides in the body's nerve cells. When reactivated, it causes blisters or raised, red spots on the skin. Typically, this rash is preceded by a fever lasting 2 to 3 days accompanied by a burning irritation or sensitivity of the skin that has been compared to severe sunburn. In approximately 5 days, the rash turns into blisters and then in another 3 days or so the yellow lesions surface, then dry up, crust over and gradually drop off. The sores hurt, itch and can cause much discomfort and often a small, pitted scar on the skin. Normally, shingles appears on one side of the body, most often on the stomach under the ribs leading to the navel. Sometimes the disease affects the lower part of the body or the upper half of the face on one side.

Even as the lesions heal, pain remains in about 5 percent of the cases. Because the virus damages the affected nerves, painful impulses can affect a person with shingles for a long time after an outbreak has subsided. This post-shingles condition is called post-viral or herpetic neuralgia and affects about one-third of PWS (people with shingles). Those past age 50 are more likely to experience HVZ episodes accompanied by post-herpetic nerve pain. This pain can be severe and last for months or even years. However, shingles is not considered contagious, but a person with shingles can pass on the original virus, possibly causing the recipient to come down with a case of chickenpox.

Preliminary research shows that giving older people a stronger form of the chicken pox vaccine used for children can boost the type of immunity believed necessary to hold the virus in check. A vaccine for shingles is expected to be available in 2006 or 2007.

**Suggested Alternative Treatments:**

- Vitamins C and E and citrus bioflavonoids are important to effectively managing shingles. Suggested dosages: vitamin C: 2,000-3,000 mg; citrus bioflavonoids:

1g and vitamin E : 400-1,600 I.U. (taken before meals). A study conducted 50 years ago found that participants received substantial relief from intravenous doses of large amounts of vitamin C over the course of 3 to 5 days. Some doctors provide in-office intravenous services.

- Vitamin $B_{12}$, which plays an important role in nerve function and maintaining nerve insulation (the protective myelin sheath) can not only shorten the duration of shingles but one physician believes it helps relieve pain better than anything now known. A study conducted in India found $B_{12}$ injections relieved pain, healed the blisters, and eliminated the pain associated with post-herpetic neuralgia. Injections are considered more efficient than supplements and typically are administered by physicians. Since B vitamins work together, take B complex (50-100 mg) and extra folic acid together with the $B_{12}$ shots.
- Bromelain (the active enzyme found in fresh pineapple) and pancreatin have shown to be effective anti-inflammatories. Suggested dosages: pancreatin: 500-1,000 mg 3 times daily before meals; bromelain: 500 mg 3 times daily on an empty stomach.

## Homeopathy

- *Ranunculus bulbous 6X*, 4 times daily (then when symptoms subside take as need for pain) for intense itching or when blisters are tightly grouped or appear on the trunk of the body.
- *Arsenicum album 30X*, 2 times daily for 2 to 3 days at the onset and when severe burning sensation or feelings of coldness are present. Blisters typically appear clear and watery. If burning sensation persists, then switch to 12C formulation, 2 to 3 times daily.

- *Hypericum perforatum 30X* is excellent for nerve pain and symptoms of burning and tingling along the affected area. Take 2 to 3 times daily as needed.

### Herbs

- Calendula-based creams may help ease itching; and creams containing capsaicin (cayenne pepper) can help relieve pain. The prescription drug Zovirax and topicals containing capsaicin should be used only after all the shingle blisters have disappeared. Do not apply to active blisters. A patch containing 5 percent lidocaine called Lidoderm, also treats post herpetic neuralgia. Because it is applied to the skin, it has less risk of side effects than pain medications taken in pill form. It is available by prescription only.

### Topical Treatment

- A warm bath with a handful of cornstarch or colloidal oatmeal mixed in may soothe the skin and help with sleep. Caution: The bottom of the tub may be slippery—be careful getting in and out of the tub.

### Aromatherapy

- Mix together 3 drops of Roman chamomile and 1 drop of lavender or rose. Add 2 tablespoons of carrier oil (canola or safflower oil) and apply 2-4 times a day. Or mix 3 drops of Melissa, 3 drops lavender, 2 drops bergamot, and 2 drops tea tree oil in a bowl; add 2 cups of water. Then dip a washcloth in mixture, wring out, and apply to lesions 2-4 times daily.

In addition, a regular practice of hatha yoga, qigong and meditation supplemented by massage also is very helpful for this condition. Get as much rest as possible.

*Avoid*: Medicines containing acetaminophen are not recommended for pain relief as these OTC drugs can prolong the outbreak. Also, stay away from chocolate.

## Canker Sores

Since they occur in the mouth, canker sores often are confused with cold sores because they also are irritating and painful. However, there are specific differences in how they appear, what causes them, and where they appear in the mouth. Cold sores appear in clusters of tiny blisters on the lips and sometimes on the gums. Canker sores tend to be smaller, crater-like lesions occurring singly or in clusters on the inside of the lips and cheeks as well as the gums and tongue. They begin a reddish small lump or swelling. Eventually the mound bursts leaving the ruptured sores covered with a white or yellow membrane. Healing time ranges from 10 to 21 days.

Cold sores or HSV-1 are contagious; canker sores are not. An estimated 56 million Americans get canker sores, with 10 to 40-year-olds as the most susceptible.

Causes of canker sores vary widely, although the specific cause has yet to be pinned down. The most cited reasons canker sores appear are because of food sensitivities, the foods most often involved are:

- Chocolate and nuts (especially walnuts)
- Fresh citrus, particularly oranges and pineapple
- Strawberries
- Tomato (fresh and cooked)
- Eggplant
- Colas and teas, especially the black variety including decaf

Frequent outbreaks also are attributed a deficiency in vitamin $B_{12}$, folic acid, zinc or iron, or a combination of these dietary supplements.

Blood tests can assist with pinpointing vitamin deficiencies as well as food allergies or sensitivities. Keeping a food diary also is helpful in determining which foods trigger outbreaks.

Other causes for canker sores include stress, heredity, menstruation, injury, fever, impaired immunity, Crohn's disease, or a body out of balance, usually too acidic. Ted Grassbart, Ph.D., a Harvard Medical School psychologist, sees a specific link between emotional stress and recurrences. He has found the most common psychological triggers are stress related to financial and sexual problems. And difficulty in expressing anger can also contribute to the appearance of canker sores.

Clinically speaking, some researchers think there is a link between hemolytic streptococcus bacteria and canker sores (as there is with stomach ulcers), with the sores a result of a hypersensitive reaction to the bacteria.

Physical stress on mouth tissues from biting the inside of the cheek, a swipe from a hard-bristled toothbrush, or dental anesthesia also can trigger a rash of canker sores. Since light and air don't easily reach the inside of the sides of the mouth, such injuries are prone to infection, and healing can be slow and tedious. Canker sores can tend to be seasonal, with outbreaks occurring more frequently in winter and spring.

The medical name for canker sores is aphthous stomatitis and they are not considered a sign of mouth cancer.

## Suggested Alternative Treatments

To prevent canker sores, eat more foods rich in vitamin C, such as broccoli, cantaloupe, and red peppers. Try eating more salads, raw onions and yogurt. Eliminate acidic foods such as citrus fruits, cereal grains and foods containing refined sugars from your diet.

Avoid commercial toothpastes and mouthwashes that contain the ingredient SLS (sodium laurel sulfate). Instead use baking soda to brush your teeth and warm salt water to rinse your mouth. Follow with a rinse of warm water with a sprinkle of dissolved sea salt, table salt, or Epsom salts. Repeat this rinse several times during the day.

Also refrain from chewing gum and tobacco and lozenges.

***To reduce pain:*** First, rinse your mouth with one teaspoonful of 3 percent hydrogen peroxide diluted in a small amount of water. Then take an acidophilus capsule, pierce it, and sprinkle a small amount on the sore. Or dab a small amount of yogurt containing live cultures. Repeat every 10-15 minutes for an hour; repeat procedure in the evening. A dab of calendula or myrrh tincture applied with a cotton swab a couple of times a day also may speed the healing process.

## Homeopathy:

Suggested dose is formulation 30X taken 3 times daily.

- *Mercurius vivus* can help at the first sign of lesions or when they appear ulcerated on the gum and tongue.
- *Borax* is indicated when there are small painful ulcers that feel hot in the mouth and may bleed while eating.

- *Mercuris Sol* if there is metallic taste in the mouth and larger, grayish ulcers. Bleeding gums also may be present.
- *Natrum Sulph* for blister-like sensitive, painful ulcers.

## Herbs

- Myrrh in tincture form is the preferred topical remedy. It possesses both astringent and healing properties.
- Pure wheat germ oil or vitamin E obtained by piercing a capsule containing the vitamin and dabbing some directly or on a cotton swab directly on the ulcer.
- Cajeput oil cools and heals sores.
- Clove oil numbs inflamed tissue and relieves pain.

## Topical Treatments

Quantum Health Formulas, who pioneered lysine-based products for herpes relief, now offers two products to relieve the mouth and canker sore discomfort and aid healing. *Canker Cover* is a tablet-like patch, made from edible ingredients, that offers protection as well as pain relief. The product works by sticking to the canker sore and dissolves into a protective film that seas and ulcer from food, drink and accidental contact from the tongue and teeth. Coverage is reported to last at least 8 hours. Canker Cover tabs are mint-flavored and contain menthol and beta carotene as well as other ingredients. Quantum Formulas also offers Canker Care+, a gel solution to coat sores with a soft applicator brush. It contains 14 ingredients including menthol, clove oil, lysine, aloe vera, tea tree oil, licorice and propolis.

## Kitchen and OTC Remedies

- Hold an antacid tablet such as a *Rolaid* against the ulcer until it dissolves.
- *Milk of Magnesia* and *Benadryl* (diphenhydramine) Liquid. Combine one teaspoonful of each and apply 4 to 6 times a day to relieve pain. Spit out mixture after each use.
- *Gly-Oxide* is a gentle, over-the-counter remedy often prescribed by dentists to cleanse and soothe oral wounds. The product's main ingredient is 10% carbamide peroxide.

## Painful Corners of the Mouth

Inflamed open cracks that appear in the corners of the mouth can often be cleared up with regular doses of vitamin $B_2$ (riboflavin). These fissures are most caused by stress and improper diet.

# Resources

## Books

### For Feeling and Living Better

Burns, David, M.D. *Feeling Good: The New Mood* Therapy. New York, NY: Penguin Putnam, 1999

Carlson, Richard, Ph.D. Easier Than You Think...because life doesn't have to be so hard: The Small Changes that Add Up to a World of Difference. San Francisco: Harper, 2005

___________. *Don't Sweat the Small Stuff. . .and it's all small stuff*. New York: Hyperion Press, 1997

Easwaran, Eknath. *Take Your Time*: Finding Balance in a Hurried World, Tomales, CA: Nilgiri Press, 1994

___________. *Strength in the Storm: Creating Calm in Difficult Times*. Tomales, CA: Nilgiri Press, 2005

Hobbs, Christopher. *Stress & Natural Healing*. Loveland, CO: Interweave Press, 1997

Groves, Dawn. *Stress Reduction for Busy People.* San Rafael, CA: New World Library, 2004

Jahnke, Roger O.M.D. *The Healer Within: Using Traditional Chinese Techniques to Release Your Body's Own Medicine*. New York, NY: Harper Collins, 1997

Jahnke, Roger O.M.D. *The Healing Promise of Qi: Creating Extraordinary Wellness Through Qigong and Tai Chi*. New York, NY: McGraw Hill, 2001

Luskin, Fred Dr. and Pelletier, Kenneth Dr. *Stress Free for Good*. San Francisco: Harper, 2005

St. James, Elaine. *Simply Your Life: 100 Ways to Slow Down and Enjoy the Things that Really Matter*. New York: Hyperion, 1994.

__________ . *Living the Simple Life*. New York: Hyperion, 1996.

Weil, M.D., Andrew, *8 Weeks to Optimum Health*, New York, NY: Ballantine
Books, 1998

__________ . *Eating Well For Optimum Health: The Essential Guide to Bringing Health and Pleasure Back to Eating*. Perennial Currents, 2001

__________ . *Spontaneous Healing: How to Discover and Embrace Your Body's Natural Ability to Maintain and Heal Itself*, New York, NY: Ballantine Books, 2001

## *Diet and Recipes*

Colbin, Anne Marie. *Food and Healing*, New York: Ballantine 1986.

Gittleman, Ann Louise Gittleman, M.S., C.N.S. *Get the Sugar Out: 501 Simple Ways to Get the Sugar Out of Any Diet*. New York: Crown Trade Paperbacks, 1996

_____________. *Your Body Knows Best: The Revolutionalry Eating Plan that Helps You Achieve Your Optimal Weight and Energy Level for Life*. New York: Pocket Books, 1997

Haigh, Charlotte. *The Top 100 Immunity Boosters: 100 Recipes to Keep Your Immune System Fighting*. Duncan Baird Publishers, 2005

Turner, Kristina. *The Self-Healing Cookbook: A Macrobiotic Prime for Healing Body, Mind and Moods with Whole, Natural Foods.* Grass Valley, CA: Earthtones Press, 2002.

## *Yoga and Meditation*

Davich, David. 8 Minute Meditation: Quiet Your Mind; Change Your Life. New York, NY: Berkeley Publishing Group, 2004

Easwaran, Eknath. *Meditation: A Simple 8-point Program for Translating Spiritual Ideals into Daily Life.* Tomales, CA: Nilgiri Press, 1991

Groves, Dawn. *Yoga for Busy People.* San Rafael, CA: New World Library, 1995

__________. *Meditation for Busy People.* San Rafael, CA: New World Library, 1993

Iyengar, B.K.S. Yoga: The Path to Holistic Health. London: Dorling Kindersley Adult, 2001

Lasater, Judith, Ph.D., P.T. *Relax and Renew: Restful Yoga for Stressful Times..* Berkeley, CA: Rodmell Press, 1995

Zinn, Jon Kabat. *Where Ever You Go, There You Are: Mindfulness Meditation in Everyday Life.* New York: Hyperion, *1994.*

## *Audio & Video Tapes*

*Accessible Yoga for Every Body*
*Yoga for the Yoga at Heart*
*Sitting Fit*
Susan Winter Ward, instructor
www. ogaheart.com

*Essentials of Qigong*
*Chi Kung: Awakening and Mastering the Medicine*
Roger Jahnke, O.M.D.
www.healerwithin.com
www.feeltheqi.com

*Qigong: Beginning Practice with Francesco & Daisy Lee Garripoli*
www.gaiam.com
877-989-6321

Jon Kabat-Zinn's *Mindfulness Meditation Practice Tapes*
www.mindfulnesstapes.com

## *Mail Order Sources*
### *Supplements, Herbs, and Topical Remedies*

**Diamond-Herpanacine Associates**
(Herpanacine)
145 Willow Grove Ave. Suite 1
Glenside, PA 19038
888-467-4200
215-542-2981
email: herpana@aol.com
www.diamondformulas.com

**Ancient Way Acupuncture & Herbs**
905 Main St. #409
Klamath Falls, OR 97601
541-884-6377
email: Kevin@ancientway.com
www.ancientway.com

**Enzymatic Therapy**
www.enzy.com
800-783-2286

**East Earth Trade Winds**
(Chinese herbs, patent formulas; consultations available)
www.eastearthherb.com
800-258-6878

**The Essential Oil Company**
www.essentialoil.com
800-729-5912

**Homeopathy Overnight**
(Extensive selection of homeopathic single and combination remedies)
www.homeopathyovernight.com
1-800-ARNICA-3

**i-herb.com**
(Large selection of discounted dietary supplements, herbs and personal care products)
www.i-herb.com
888-792-0028

**Life's Vigor.com**
(Wide selection of natural products, including Herpanacine, at competitive prices)
www.lifesvigor.com
661-589-1818

**Morningstar Health.com**
(Chinese patent formulas, dietary supplements)
www.morningstarhealth.com

**Nature's Sunshine Products**
(Comprehensive selection of quality vitamins, herbs, Chinese herbs and personal care products)
www.naturesshine.com
800-453-1422

**Quantum Health Formulas**
(Lysine formulas, dietary supplements and topicals for herpes and canker sores)
www.quantumhealth.com
800-448-1448

## Testing

**University of Washington Virology Lab**
http://depts.washington.edu/herpes/
For testing with the Western Blot, most accurate blood test for detecting herpes, have your health care provider call 206-598-6066 to request the HSV type-specific serology information packet.

For the information on the location of specific labs that use HerpeSelect Elisa Kits and HerpeSelect Immunoblot Kit, call 800-445-4032.

**National Herpes Hotline**
**919-361-8488**

**Centers for Disease Control and Prevention**
**National STD Hotline**
**1-800-227-8922**

# *Notes*

# *Notes*

*Notes*

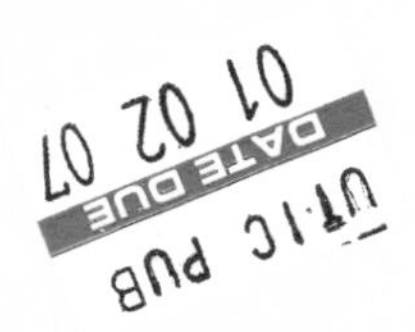




Printed in the United States
51414LVS00002B/36